Unruly Curls

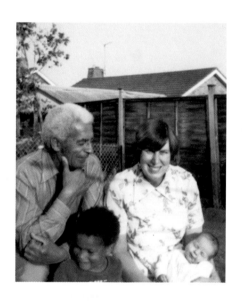

I DEDICATE THIS BOOK TO MY GRANDPARENTS,
JUNE AND ERIC ACKLAND. THEIR LOVE
AND ENDURING MIXED-MATRIMONY IS AN
INSPIRATION AND I AM PROUD.

Unruly Curls

How to manage, style and love your curly hair

MICHAEL PRICE

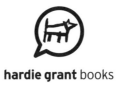

hardie grant books

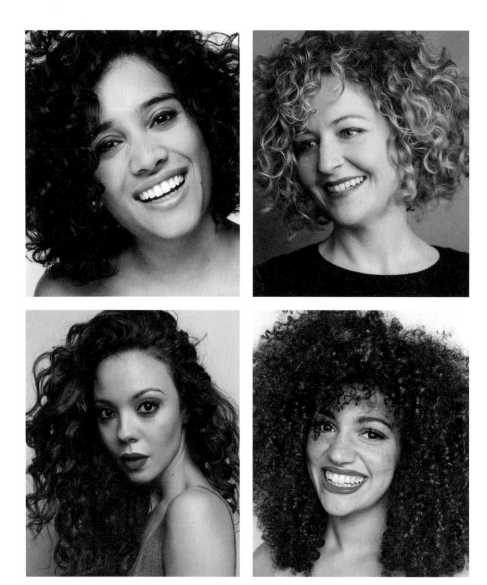

Contents

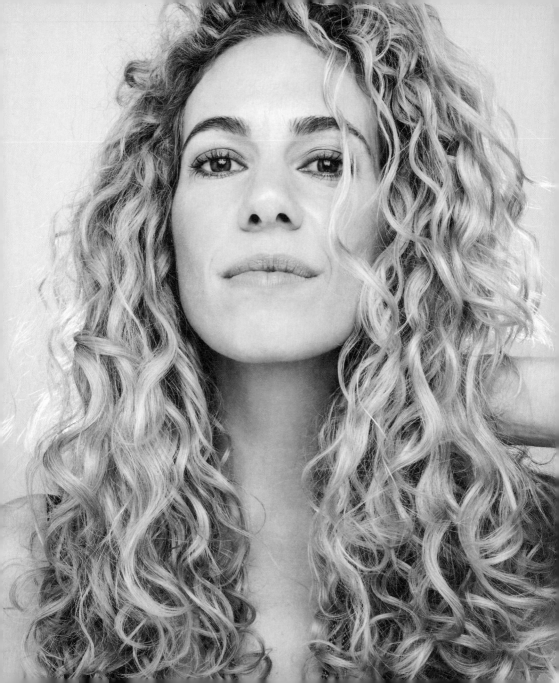

Spirals, corkscrews, twists and waves...
it's time to celebrate your unruly hair.

Introduction

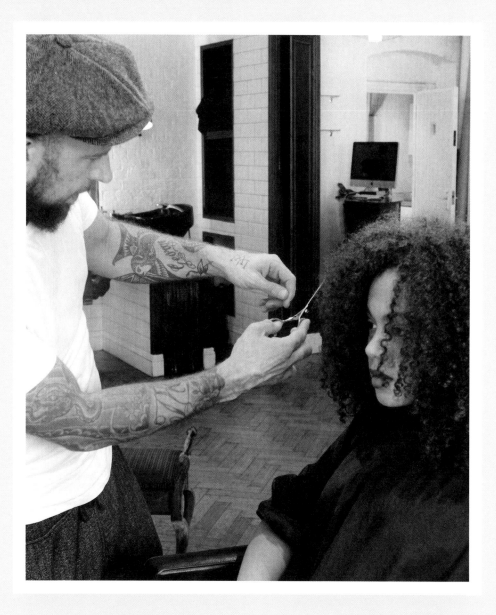

Curls and me

————

Unruly: disobedient, unmanageable, uncontrollable, stubborn, disorderly, riotous.

If you've ever thought this about your hair, you're not alone. It was certainly the case with mine growing up, which was one of the reasons why I became a curly hair specialist.

I come from an ethnically diverse family and I'm very proud of my roots. My grandfather probably came from Kenya, of East African descent, and it's from him that my family's curly hair originates. When I was a kid, this was quite unusual. I was white-skinned, with pretty Afro-like hair, so I both got abuse for my 'fro, and also heard people being openly racist in front of me, with no idea that my brother and grandfather were black and my mother mixed-race. Not easy.

As I grew up, however, my hair and its appearance became more crucial to my success with girls in particular. My confidence took a hit after an incident when a girl I fancied made a comment to my brother, asking whether I was his 'little sister'. This caused me to have long-lasting insecurities about my appearance that extended throughout my teenage life. I experimented with styles that worked for straight hair and by my mid-teens I had started to try growing it out, and duly suffered much more than my fair share of hair disasters. Overall, I lost faith in hairdressers. I tried my luck with Afro salons and was told they couldn't cut my type of hair. I tried expensive salons and they too seemed unable to cope. Nobody knew how to style hair like mine.

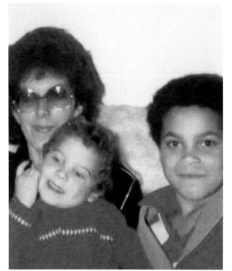
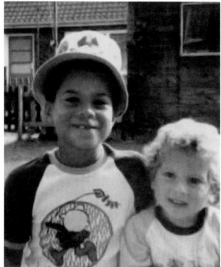
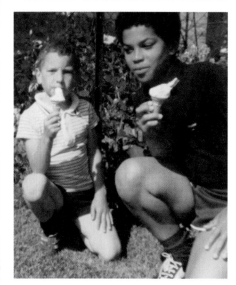
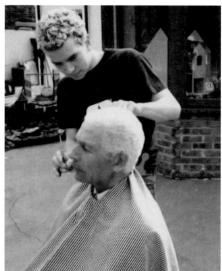

'If you could manage your mother's hair, you could master anyone's!'

Long before I took to the trade of hairdressing myself, I had already gathered a sense of what worked and what didn't. I was 13 years old when I first talked about hairdressing as a career option. My mother, whose mixed Afro-Euro hair is the true definition of difficult, encouraged it, no doubt so that I might become a live-in helping hand with her own daily hair struggle. The hairdresser that cared for our family's hair at home once said, 'If you could manage your mother's hair, you could master anyone's!'

I attribute my curly hair ability to being able to practise on my mother's hair. Her hair was normal to me from birth. She maxed out her hair boldly, in full celebration of its powerful impact on top of her six-foot frame. It morphed in shape through the decades, never failing to act as a beacon of her confidence and personality. Although it was familiar and similar to mine, I never thought I'd end up cutting it. Her eagerness to find a solution to manage it led her to enlist my help at the first word of me announcing hairdressing as a career option. I remember sitting and watching her hair being done when I was a child and gradually as I got older I started thinking, 'I could do that.' At the time I started cutting her hair, I was totally unaware that I would one day be able to appreciate how uniquely different and difficult hers is compared to the many thousands of heads of hair I have worked with since.

Her hair was so resilient to any kind of styling effort and had a density to it that I have rarely, if ever, seen since. Developing the skills to work with my mother's hair, without becoming overwhelmed by its mass, was essential if anything was to be done with it. Doing her hair played an essential part in how I work now. Not being intimidated when a client with kinky, curly or wavy hair walks in is the first step to earning trust and confidence.

Now, 25 years deep into my hairdressing career, I remain baffled by what I consider to be the widespread lack of training and understanding of curly hairdressing throughout the industry. My salon, Unruly Curls, located in London's Notting Hill, is vastly oversubscribed, with a lengthy waiting time for an appointment. While I have enjoyed years of being in demand as a curly hair specialist, profiting from my industry's neglect and failure to meet the needs of curly-haired people, this is not all that I feel I can contribute. Helping one person at a time is rewarding, but limited. I want to share my professional knowledge and skill throughout this book, and help those with curly hair enjoy a better relationship with their tresses!

11

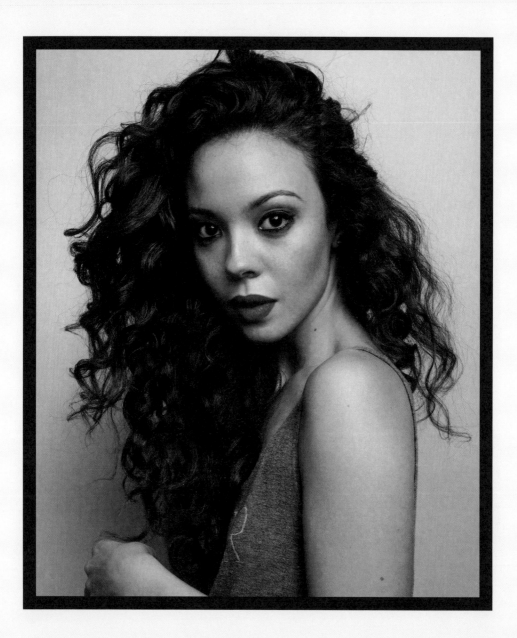

CURL CASE: IANA

ETHNICITY: ERITREAN AND ITALIAN

My hair has always been an odd and ambivalent companion. In my earliest youth, I covered it in a towel to pretend that the triangular cloud on my head and matching rat's tail was actually a straight, long, flowing Disney dream. As I left Brazil for Asia and was met by women whose hair, unlike mine, fully embraced its gravitational potential, the scent of burning hair became part of my aura. By the time I was 16, most people thought I had naturally straight hair and I reveled in my little secret as my curls made their brief cameo once a week, in the mirror, before they were duly squashed into submission.

It wasn't until adolescence wore away and my aspirations outgrew the hair on my head and the feeling of non-acceptance centred around it that I allowed my natural hair to grow untouched. What grew seemed to echo my heritage and personality perfectly and summoned sighs of relief from my parents in tandem, who assured me that Botticelli had once had dreams about hair like mine.

Today, my time and energy is focused on taking care of my patients, on family, on painting, reading and dancing. Left to its own devices, my hair has somehow become everything it was always meant to be – an insulating, vibrant, unique representation of me.

Knowledge is power, so if you want
to reclaim control over your hair, you need
to know what it's made of.

What is Hair?

CHAPTER 1

16

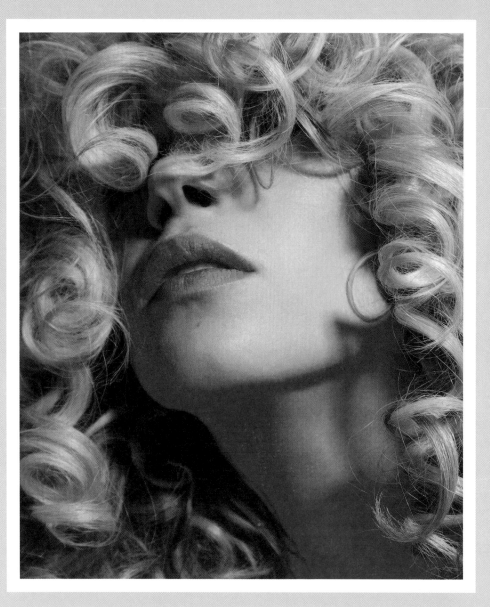

Hair: the inside story

———————————

While it's not essential to know exactly what hair is, it's helpful to consider its basic structure in order to understand how to look after it. Learning more about your hair is the first step on your journey towards curl revolution!

Hair is a fibrous strand made mostly of a protein called keratin. It covers areas of the body susceptible to heat loss and provides thermal insulation. It helps to block ultraviolet rays, and also helps keep us cool us by wicking away sweat.

Looking at hair up close immediately gives a greater sense of its strengths and weaknesses. The hair on our heads is incredibly fast-growing and hard-wearing compared to the hair on the rest of our bodies. Viewed under a microscope, healthy hair is remarkably unevenly textured.

Alongside each hair's root is a tiny muscle that lifts the hair from the scalp, helping to regulate body temperature by creating a controlled thermal barrier. Each follicle has a sebaceous gland that secretes our own natural protection from bacteria, called sebum. This also hydrates hair, freeing it from knotting, and helps reduce static attraction of micro-atmospheric particles. Sebum has such a vital role; it should not be looked down on as grease, but should be considered vital to the health of our hair and scalp.

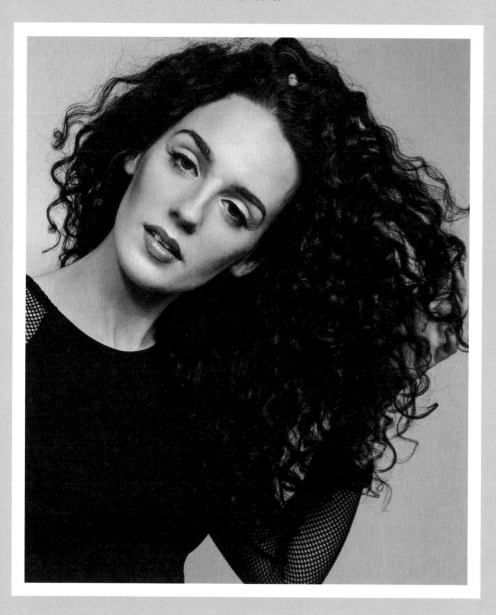

So you have curly hair...

The majority of people with curly hair wrongly consider themselves to be in a minority group. However, studies have concluded that more people have curly rather than straight hair. Many curly-haired people fail to appreciate their hair and have a negative attitude towards it. Too many hairdressers fail to see where they are getting it wrong and miss the fact that a huge percentage of people feel inadequately served.

Many hairdressers are still busy straightening curly or wavy hair, turning it into something that is easier for them to control or manage, often ignorantly assuming that straighter hair is more desirable or 'polished'. This results in haircuts that only work after hours of damaging heat styling, as opposed to cuts that work with the natural curl of the hair and look their best when dried naturally or with minimum heat (see pages 42–47 for tips on drying your hair).

When we don't feel great, this can often be reflected by our hair. The hair on our heads is a relatively non-critical part of our bodies, so when we are ill, or even severely emotionally stressed, our bodies redirect the energy for the production of hair-building cells towards fighting the sickness, or whatever else it is challenged with. This can lead to people getting trapped in a vicious cycle where their hair looks lacklustre, but they feel too rundown to improve its appearance, which in turn makes them feel even worse.

In today's world, many people view their hair as a rather challenging project, requiring the investment of time, money and effort in order for us to look healthy, and thus more attractive. For a curly-haired person, even more time and effort is required, as something as minor as a sweatshirt being pulled on or off can render curls a mess. Getting a decent haircut is a mission, and despite the fact that we have seen footage of men walking on the moon, many well-paid professional hairdressers simply haven't got a damn clue about how to dry curly hair without making it straight, let alone how to cut it well.

It's amazing how much a curly-haired person's experience can be changed for the better with just a good stylist and the right information. There are just a few simple things you need to learn in order to gain control over the chaos of curls, get a reasonable haircut, and make your curls look better on day two after washing. I hope to bust the myth that curly hair always has to be a struggle.

Those with curly hair can also face the extra challenge due to the perception that their hair is not suitable for an executive role or a corporate environment, believing that it can suggest that they are disorganised, chaotic, messy, bubbly, a pushover, or even a bit crazy. In reality, well-cared-for curls worn with conviction are likely to enhance your natural beauty and will let it shine through, giving you real presence; you will convey vitality, creativity and self-confidence.

20

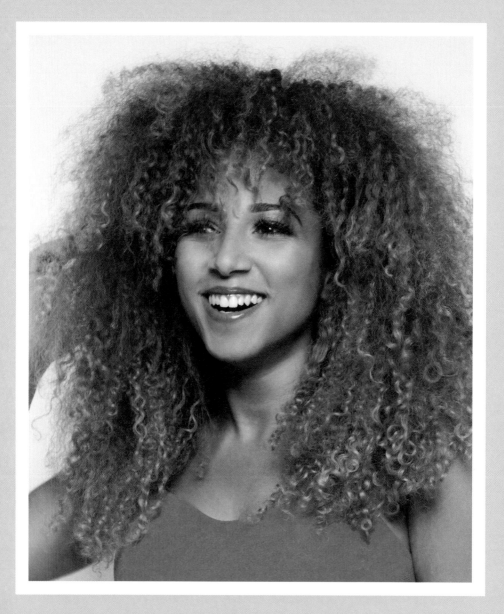

Curl revolution

Right now, in my cosmopolitan home city of London, curly hair is enjoying a revival. It should be no wonder that after years of multiculturalism and with the vast ethnic mix it boasts, London's diverse, modern society is striving for greater equality, understanding and acceptance. This is aided massively by social media and supported by a new generation of youth that know nothing other than globalisation and multiculturalism. It is seen as high time by those that have suffered early mornings to fight against their curls in an attempt to be more in line with the perceived standard of what is beautiful. More and more online groups for those with curly hair are being launched and their followings grow rapidly as the curl revival kicks into a higher gear. Many people now use social media to publicly document their transitions back to their true identities as being naturally curly-haired.

Transitioning

Transitioning has become the buzzword for the process of nurturing damaged, less curly or straightened hair back to healthy, natural curls. Curly roots that suddenly turn into straight ends are a very unnatural look to pull off. This is actually the opposite of how hair is naturally: straighter or at least looser at the root and curlier toward the end. Common causes of the related damage include chemical relaxing, straightening, excessive heat styling, twisting, over-processing with colour, or bleach. The transition back to

having curls takes time. Even a year in, people can find themselves with only a few inches of thick, healthy new hair at the root and many more inches of straight, lifeless hair towards the tips.

It's a huge challenge as a hairdresser to be confronted with this situation. The only real options are either to accept that the hair must undergo a long growing-out process until a decent haircut can be achieved or, at the extreme end, to cut off all the damaged hair for a dramatically shorter style. Although many people feel very liberated when they do cut it short, I totally understand why some have a strong fear of losing so much hair in one haircut – hair is a huge part of our identities.

That's why I hope that this book will give people the power to reclaim their hair and, in turn, themselves!

This book and you

Like many others, you may be in transition back to curly hair – and want to know and be reassured that this transition will be successful for you. Or you may be someone who just knows you could manage your unruly tresses better. With greater knowledge about your hair, its care, cutting, products, styling and more, you can be reassured that your unruly curls can become a crowning glory that speaks volumes about the confident, successful person you are.

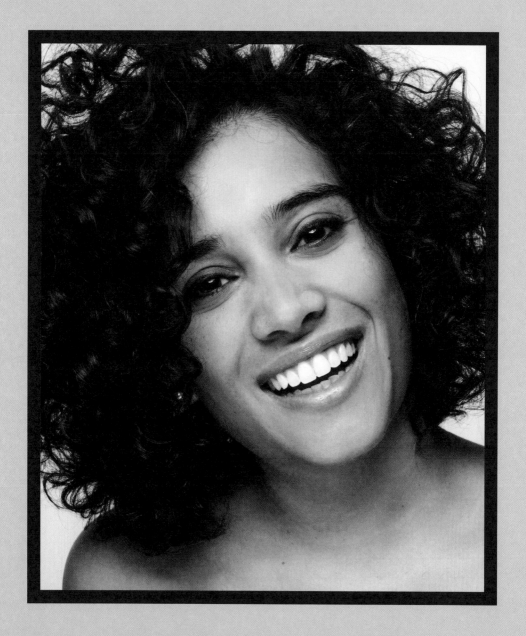

CURL CASE: ANJULI

ETHNICITY: INDIAN

It starts when we are children, and all the straight-haired girls wear their hair down. But ours is always tied up. It's unruly, so our practical mums want it up and out of the way. Then comes puberty. We experiment with wearing it down. But it's frizzy. I mean, *really* frizzy. We don't know how to use products. We stick out like a sore thumb in all the class photos. So we start straightening it. Trying to tame the unruliness; trying to fit in. But on a humid day, or if it rains, it goes right back to being a wild mishap.

I first learned to embrace my curls when I was 19 and moved to Kuwait to teach kindergarten. After so many years of tying it up and straightening it, it's safe to say that my hair was pretty damaged. In a country that covers its hair, I rebelled and started to wear mine down. Slowly, over the months, something remarkable happened. The curls started forming in the same pattern. The frizz started turning into bounce. The bristle texture started to turn soft. One year later I had a beautiful head of long, thick, dark curls. I felt like I was reborn, with renewed confidence. I was a girl with beautiful curls and, more importantly, I realised my hair was a representation of who I was inside. The fun-loving, carefree, soft, strong, resilient me.

Ask any girl about her curls, and she will get emotional. After all, it is the most liberated manifestation of her soul.

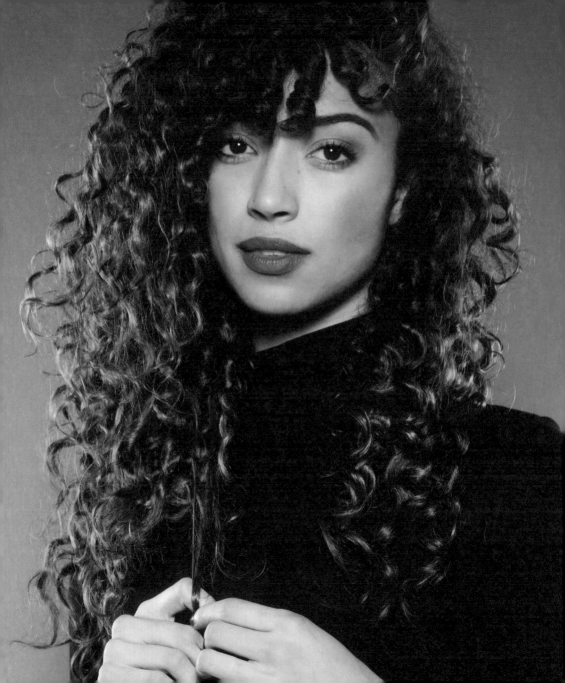

Now you've embraced your beautiful curly hair,
understanding it and knowing how to care for it
will help you get the best from your curls.

Curl Care

CHAPTER 2

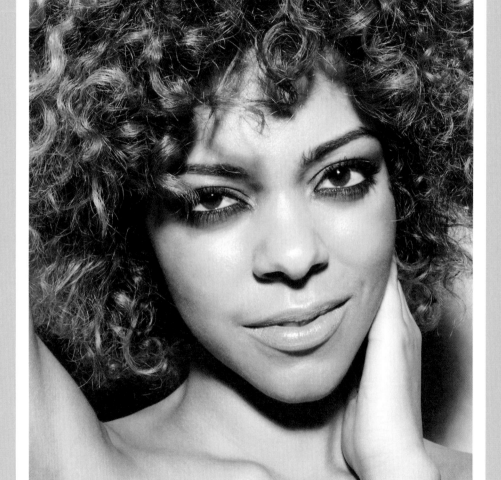

Curl types

___

So your curls are unruly, but what else do you know about them?

Hair can be classified into four main types: straight, wavy, curly and kinky. If you're reading this, you probably don't belong to the first group!

Wavy hair lies between straight and curly. It can be resistant to styling and prone to frizz.

Curly hair has more definite, S-shaped curls. Many of my clients have this hair type, which is considered the most temperamental. But don't worry – follow the advice in this book and your life will be made easier.

Kinky hair tends to be fine and fragile, made up of tightly coiled curls in a zigzag pattern. It requires delicate handling and tons of moisture to stay healthy.

Even across the scalp, hair differs, and over time it can change a lot in colour and shape.

How do I look after my curls?

**Keeping your beautiful curls happy and healthy
is simple if you follow a few basic pointers.**

WASHING If you have long or thick curly hair, a powerful shower will help a great deal. Using a jug to rinse hair is okay, but will take much longer. Start by fully soaking your hair from root to tip. Shake the excess water out of your hair and spread a small amount of shampoo across wet hands.

The main aim of washing is to clean your hair at the roots and maintain good scalp health. Focus on the roots rather than the lengths to avoid drying out your hair. Wash with small, circular motions using your fingertips, avoiding scrubbing aggressively with your nails, which will irritate your scalp. If you select a strong shampoo, washing will take less time. If you go for a gentler shampoo you will need to work harder in place of the chemicals. Don't go overboard, or your hair will become overly stressed.

CO-WASHING Co-washing is a fantastic option if you find your hair dry and difficult to hydrate. It is simply doing away with shampoo and using conditioner to wash your hair instead. There are products marketed specifically as co-wash or conditioning cleansers. These are intended to be the missing link between a shampoo, which typically will dry some curly hair out, and straight-up conditioner, which can often leave hair heavy or feeling clogged. A co-wash will both cleanse your hair and condition it at the same time. I encourage my clients to try shampooing much less often, focusing their efforts on how, rather than with what. To co-wash, simply wet your hair, and use conditioner as a shampoo. It won't lather, so it will feel strange, but get stuck in and rinse well and you will find your hair can feel just as clean as with shampoo.

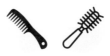

COMBING V. BRUSHING

There is a big difference between when you should use a brush instead of a comb. See pages 78–79 to find out more.

29

CONDITIONING Apply conditioner to your hair and do not cover your scalp too much. Be careful when combing through your hair and don't allow yourself a false sense of it doing less damage. When hair is wet it has three times the elasticity of dry hair. Wet hair covered with conditioner will allow hands and combs to slip through easily, while preventing you from getting a real sense of how your hair is being pulled. A brush going through wet conditioned hair will further remove the sensation of how knotty your hair is. This means you might be likely to brush your hair much more firmly than you would if it wasn't wet or covered in conditioner, leading to greater risk of breakage and split ends. Be aware of this and be gentle at all times. Even if your hair is slippery and conditioned, make sure to comb gently to preserve those luscious locks.

DEEP CONDITIONING Although I firmly believe that hair can only be superficially made to feel repaired until the next wash, I still appreciate the benefit of deep conditioning even if it is superficial. If it assists with managing your hair and prevents further damage it is a good thing. I often negotiate with a client that is unwilling to cut away all the damaged hair by agreeing that they should invest time and effort in thoroughly hydrating it with the treatment, wrapping it when applied, allowing the heat to open up the hair's cuticle and saturate deep within. Rinsing thoroughly with cool or even cold water will cause porous hair to close up quickly, sealing some of the deep conditioner into the cavities that exist in damaged hair. Wear it naturally dried for as long as possible to give your hair time to appreciate the deep conditioner.

Products

Products fall into four main categories: washing, conditioning, styling and colouring, and the wealth of choice demonstrates that products are big business, especially for curly-haired people for whom the wash 'n' run option isn't really viable. Using a different product than your regular one can have a noticeable effect on how your hair looks, feels and smells and many people switch regularly in search of the perfect one. The creativity of manufacturers seems to be never-ending, as they strive to produce the next big thing, claiming to do all sorts of wonders for us with one new fantastic ingredient after the other. I am dubious about the bigger claims and would urge you to be wary of any self-proclaimed miracle workers!

Wet-look, firm-hold gel or mousse, and wax. These were my everything when I was a young, curly-haired boy in Kent.

SHAMPOO The shampoo you use to wash your hair and exactly how you wash your hair are equally important. Shampoos all work differently. If your shampoo is too strong, it might make your hair dry; too weak and it might be ineffective. You may need to experiment with a few good-quality shampoos (see my favourites on page 111) to find out what works for you.

A word on sulphates. Used in shampoos, sulphates are surfactants (molecules that have been engineered to attract both oil and water), hence their ability to remove oil from hair. Natural cleansing agents such as tea tree, eucalyptus and others do cleanse, but are usually less effective than ingredients such as sodium lauryl sulphate or sodium laureth sulphate. These are used in shampoos because they are effective. They are capable of washing hair very well, as long as they are used alongside other ingredients that negate their drying ability, such as conditioners.

It doesn't take much shampoo to do a good job. If possible, it's better to use less shampoo so that your hair does not suffer from build-up of product. If you gradually reduce the amount of shampoo you use, and wash with more physical effort, you won't need so much product and can even eventually replace full-strength shampoo with a mild cleanser. Gently massage your scalp and hair with your hands, using only a little shampoo but plenty of water and friction to rid it of dust, dirt and dry skin.

In the salon, we use sulphate-, mineral oil-, additive-, paraben- and silicon-free Cantu Cleansing Cream shampoo (see page 111). It is inexpensive, effective and kinder to curly hair than many available. We experiment with new shampoos all the time but also prefer to demonstrate how being minimal with shampoo can reap good results.

CONDITIONERS Conditioners are definitely a friend of curly hair, whether you use shampoo or are completely shampoo-free. They make life with curly hair much easier. The better moisturised your hair, the healthier and easier to work with it will be.

I recommend using several different conditioners: one that is cheaper and thicker to use when detangling; another that is possibly more expensive, but better at moisturising and hydrating hair for less frequent use. Find a deep conditioner that rinses out without weighing the hair down and becoming tacky, attracting dirt and suffocating the scalp.

CURL DEFINING Curl-defining products are the Holy Grail to the curly-haired person keen on controlling and maximising the beauty of their curls. Bear in mind, though, that over time those products with huge amounts of alcohol or low-grade silicones eventually build up or dry hair out.

The main characteristics I look for are products that don't flake when scrunched into the hair, and those that don't feel sticky or tacky. I find hair that is styled with a sticky product, or one that loses its ability to hold curls after being touched, rarely survives a night's sleep.

Many products that tick all the styling boxes can fail to leave curly hair shiny, but have a matte, dulling effect instead. Experiment with what suits your hair. As ever, I am a proponent of the 'less is more' approach when it comes to these products: learn how to use it, but use less of it.

OILS I am a tremendous believer in the benefit of using oil on your scalp. Not excessively, but as a way to mimic the natural functioning of your scalp's own production until you manage to achieve a good look relying solely on your own oils.

Oils such as argan, sweet almond and coconut have nutritional value and can benefit your scalp and hair as their viscosity is close to that of our own sebum, therefore helping to hydrate and lubricate it. The best thing about pure oils is that they don't contain chemicals found in many products, and the minerals and vitamins encourage hair growth.

HEAT PROTECTION There is nothing, really, that will fully protect your hair from the heat of most styling tools, as they use temperatures ranging from 90–300°C (200–570°F). You can still use these tools, but understand that any intense heat application can damage the hair over time, so my recommendation is to only use them occasionally.

31

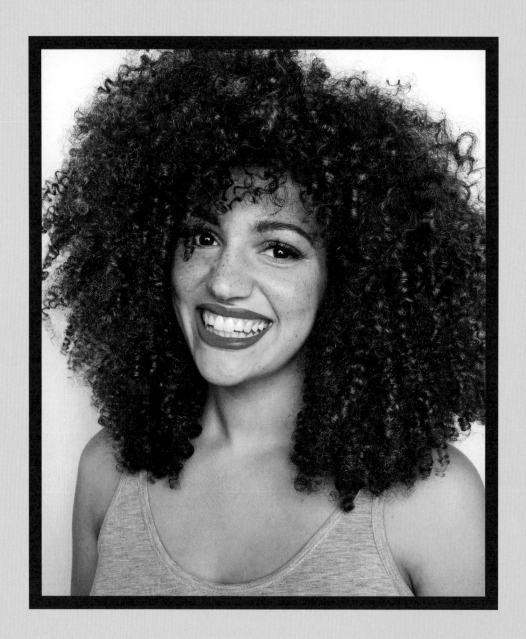

CURL CASE: TIRI

ETHNICITY: ENGLISH AND CARIBBEAN

When I was in my early teens, I really hated my curls!
I wanted long, straight hair like all my friends. Living in
Cornwall, UK, nobody in my school had curls like mine. So
after nagging my mum every day to let me relax my hair, she
finally gave in and took me to a salon in London to have it done
(in Cornwall nobody knew how to relax hair – there just wasn't
the demand for it). I came out of the salon sooooo happy...
until my roots started to come through and I had to straighten
my hair every day. My hair got very damaged and I wanted my
curls back, so I had my straightened, lifeless hair cut off. It was
a shock for a while having such short hair, but I soon got used
to it and since that day I have only ever had a trim.

I love trying out new hair products; I'm always on social media
looking at girls with similar curls to mine and buying the
products they use. I now find it exciting to embrace my curls!

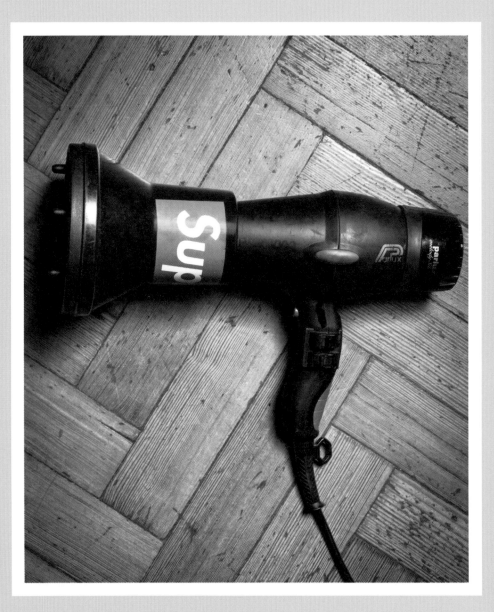

What does the damage?

———————————

Caring for curly hair should start with the mantra, 'First, do no damage'. This is easier said than done, but understanding how the choices you make could inflict damage on your curly hair will help you minimise this.

HEAT Hair is delicate, structurally complex and takes a long time to grow. For this reason, you should be extra careful when blasting it with hot air or squeezing it between hot plates!

In curly hair, the tiny structures also form a coil or wave that is dependent on the integrity of its structure being fully intact. While straight hair may appear dull, limp or brittle when it's damaged, curly hair can also change in shape after being damaged, typically becoming straighter or looser. In my opinion, the change in the curl pattern is the worst aspect of heat damage: it is rarely a uniform shape change, but rather an irregular and chaotic, frizz-forming, discombobulating effect.

Because heat can be so damaging, I recommend avoiding heat styling and instead drying hair naturally if at all possible (see pages 42–43).

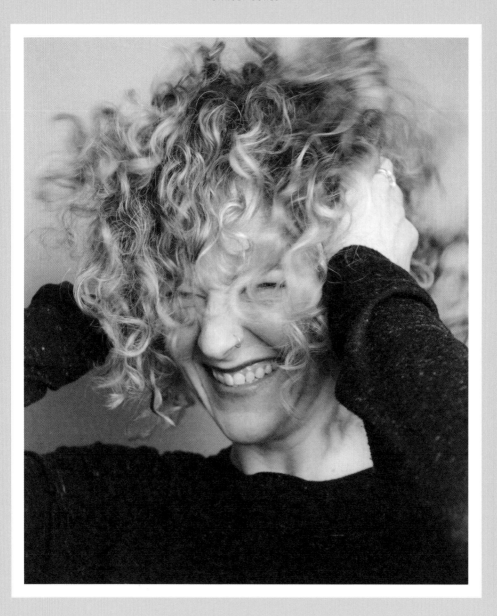

WASHING It might surprise you that simply washing your hair can lead to damage. However, if you consider that wet hair is more elastic and shampoo can be quite drying, you can imagine how hair that is parched and then stressed by a poorly executed wash can become very knotty. In the process people will often find themselves roughly untangling hair just to get the job done quickly. No matter how short on time you are, always be gentle when lathering your hair and ensure that you use shampoos and conditioners that will enrich, rather than harm, your hair (see pages 30–31).

ENVIRONMENT Something as subtle as your environment can lead to curly hair becoming damaged. Hard water is also hard on the hair. If you live in a hard water area, consider installing a water softener. Exposing yourself to too much sunlight may lighten the colour of your hair and in the process it will become more porous and difficult to manage. Consider covering your hair or using a styling product that is UV-filtering, and see pages 99–101 for summer hair tips and treatments. Take care of your hair in environments where it is likely to be exposed to lots of static and dirt, and expect it to need a little more TLC post-exposure.

OVER-TREATMENT Constant treating of hair with heavy, thick, sticky treatments will start to have an adverse effect on your curls. Hair that has excessive amounts of any product on it will start to become weighed down and even attract more dirt. The build-up of deep conditioners will also start to meddle with the fine chemistry and balance of your scalp, potentially leading to irritation. Be moderate with conditioning treatments and be sure to follow the instructions. Leaving them on way longer than recommended is not a good idea if you want to avoid a negative impact on the shape and structure of your curls.

DIET AND DEHYDRATION Your diet and water intake can have a real impact on your hair. The outer layer of hair is protected by keratin, a protein, so maintaining a high protein intake will help your hair stay strong and lustrous. Make sure you aren't deficient in iron by eating plenty of leafy greens. Consuming fatty acids will help avoid a dry scalp – try avocado, nuts or oily fish. It's imperative to stay hydrated to keep your hair in top condition. Hair cells require water to transport vitamins and minerals to the hair root, so dehydration can lead to limp, lifeless hair. Drink at least eight glasses of water a day to keep your hair hydrated and shiny.

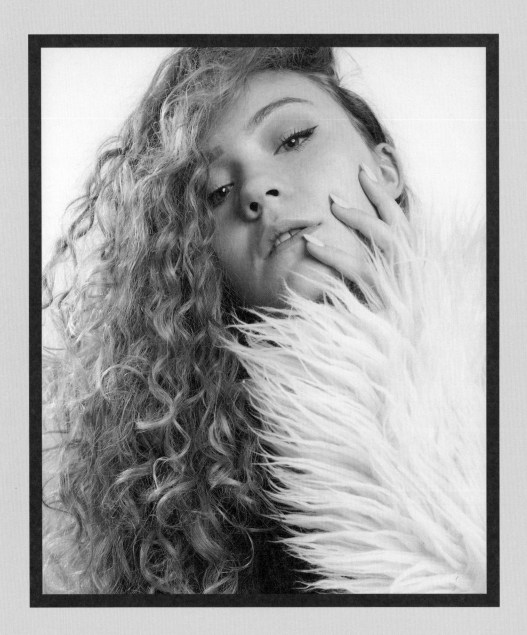

CURL CASE: ALEXANDRA

ETHNICITY: SWEDISH

I was quite a wild child, but at least my hair was well behaved… until I hit puberty and then bam! Curl explosion. I had no idea what to do and, since no one else in my family has curly hair, neither did anyone around me. I walked around with a frizzy pouf on my head for years until I met a hairdresser who told me I shouldn't even be brushing my hair. I was fairly lazy, so that suited me perfectly.

Spending hours each day straightening my hair sounds like a horrible time to me, so when I was told I would be better off not washing it for several days and never taking a brush to it, I was sold. I think curly hair adds a lot of character and makes you stand out. I'm so happy that I learnt to embrace it!

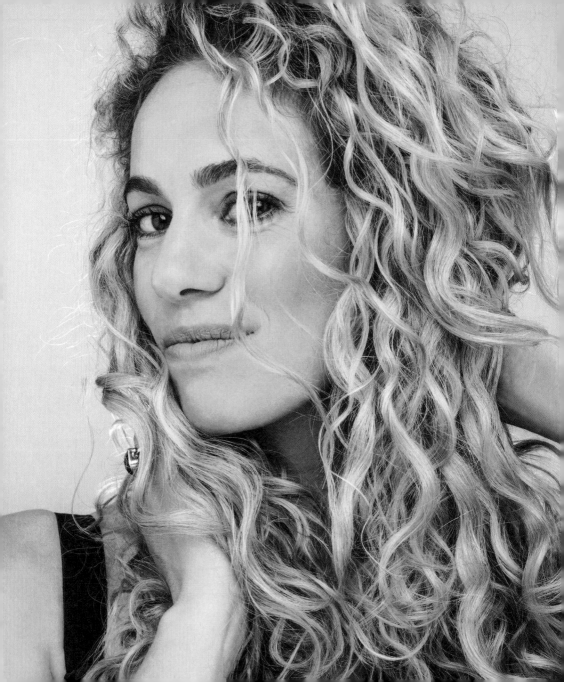

Curly hair loves being styled. It has the benefit of being all things: big, huge, chaotic, disco-fro and bouffant, or smooth, defined, pristine and sleek.

Styling Curly Hair

CHAPTER 3

Drying

___

In an ideal world, we would always leave our hair to dry naturally, but this isn't always feasible. In addition, it is often in the drying process that we can bring style to our hair, so it's worth considering how to get the best out of different methods for your curls.

42

Natural

___

Natural drying is the most essential way to learn to style your curly hair. Letting your hair dry by itself is absolutely the best, because it embraces what you already have and is the least damaging, presenting no threat at all to the health of your hair. It relies on having a decent haircut and will work best when your hair is in good condition. It requires the greatest amount of time, so factor this in before you begin.

1. For the very best natural drying result, it is important that the process begins in the bath or shower. Wash or co-wash (see page 28), then rinse well, condition your hair thoroughly and comb through, removing all tangles.

2. Using a jug of water if in the bath or the flow of the water from your showerhead, continue to rinse while keeping your hair detangled. Use your fingers at first and then just the flow of the water, allowing your hair to hang as one solid, unified, wet mass of conditioned, detangled hair down your back. The main aim is to remove the impression of the fine separation created by the comb; you want to aim for drenched, detangled hair hanging together in one beautiful, shimmering curtain.

3. Wet your hands and apply a small amount of whichever defining product you choose, coating your palms and fingers. Keep your fingers

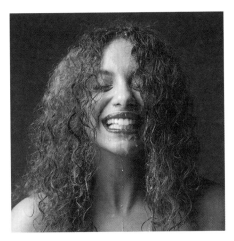
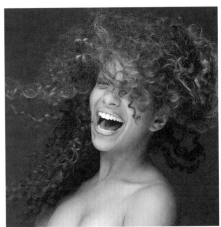

43

together throughout this process, as using them to comb through the hair will create the kind of separation you are trying to avoid.

4. Keep your head upturned, concentrating on gathering all of the ends into your hands, and scrunch the product into your hair. With much of the water still in your hair and the product on your wet hands, the product will distribute and dilute as you squelch and scrunch it through your hair, coating the mid-lengths and tips with a small amount of product. Keep doing this until your hair stops dripping. Be particularly careful not to get your fingers caught up in your hair. You are essentially scrunching and squeezing the product in at the same time as removing as much of the moisture as possible. Take great care not to pull or comb any of your hair during this step.

Grab handfuls of your hair and squeeze it by piling and gathering it in such a way as to encourage as much curl as possible. I recommend performing this stage whilst still standing over the bath or shower.

5. Now turn your head back upright without flipping it. Flipping it quickly will draw out the curl. Instead, turn your head upright and gently shake your hair side to side to get it out of your face. Your hair will be much damper at this stage compared to how it would be after towel drying, so expect it to take longer to dry. Avoid touching it as it dries and avoid going out in strong winds or driving in a car with the windows open. To speed the process along continue to scrunch it occasionally. Once your hair is dry, you will be left with beautifully bouncy, natural curls.

Diffuser

Using a diffuser is the quickest and easiest way to dry curly hair, capturing and embracing its natural texture. Going directly from the shower or bath when your hair is still soaking wet and freshly detangled will ensure a more defined finish.

1. For the best results with a diffuser, follow the steps for natural drying (pages 42–43).

2. Start diffusing your hair with your head forward, gathering your scrunched curls and gently cradling them in the diffuser. Ensuring the wind power is on a low setting will prevent frizz and help stop your hairdryer producing too high a temperature.

3. Patiently hold your hair in place. For a tighter curl hold the dryer closer to your head with your hair bunched up between your head and the diffuser; for looser curls or waves allow your hair to hang more freely. Holding the diffuser closer to your head will trap the hot air and thus will dry your hair quicker, as there is less room for the hot air to escape. Holding it further away will mean it takes longer to dry.

4. Tilting or hanging your head forward and to the sides will allow the hot air to get to the roots of your hair, which will add volume and will also dry your hair quicker. Pointing a diffuser at the side of your hair with your head upright will cause the wind and heat to bounce off the surface of your hair, unsettling the outer layer and causing frizz, while the inner layer remains wet.

44

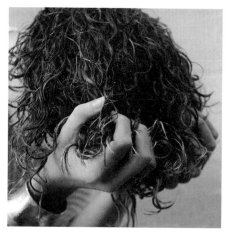

SCRUNCH YOUR HAIR WITH YOUR HANDS

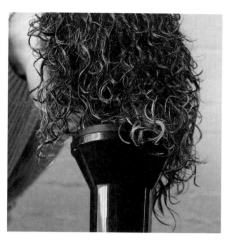

CRADLE YOUR CURLS WITH THE DIFFUSER

HELPFUL NOTES ON USING A DIFFUSER

✱ The wetter the better

The wetter your hair is when you begin using the diffuser, the more defined it will be. Typically, people towel dry their hair, then use lots of product to make it defined. By using a small amount of product on un-towel-dried hair you will achieve the same amount of definition without caking your hair in product.

✱ Patience and stillness

Think of 'the tortoise and the hare' or 'less haste, less waste'. By constantly moving the diffuser from one section to another you not only risk disturbing the curl, you will also not allow the diffuser to get to the temperature required to actually dry your hair. For most of the process it is much better to remain patient and work in a controlled manner. I advise my clients to be still and move the dryer much less until the hair is approximately 80 per cent dry, before getting involved in scrunching the hair. I sometimes outline the requirement to remain still, calm and methodical by explaining the concept as follows. If you have one cake to bake and the use of three ovens, there is little sense opening the door of one oven, allowing the heat to escape while removing it from one oven and opening the door of the next oven allowing the heat from that to escape, while placing the cake into the second oven. Basically – shut the door and leave it in to do the job. Every time you move the diffuser you are allowing the still damp hair to cool down while starting on a new section or area, which will take time to get back up to the temperature required to actually start drying it.

✱ Growth patterns and partings

Generally, a good haircut ought to be tailored to your natural parting. I typically define the parting after drying. To easily find your natural parting, flip your head forward then slowly return your head back upright, while gently shaking your head from side to side. Any attempt to define a parting with a comb will disturb your natural curl and the result of diffusing a combed section of hair will look vastly different to the rest of your uncombed curls.

✱ Timing

I recommend getting started with the diffuser as rapidly as possible after leaving the shower. The effectiveness of a diffuser is due to the drying process being conducted evenly, taking your hair from wet to dry. If you wait too long before starting to diffuse, your hair will start to dry naturally before you start drying the core of the curl clusters. The already dry outer areas will risk being over-dried, which may cause damage.

✱ Damage

Heat-styling curly hair is undoubtedly among the most common causes of damage to curly hair. Studies have concluded that hair that is routinely exposed to temperatures over 135.2°C (275°F) shows visible signs of damage. My faithful Parlux 3000 hairdryer with a diffuser attached, set to high heat and low wind, creates exactly and consistently 110°C (230°F). Take care with your hair and remember how damaging heat can be. Choose your tools well (see pages 75–83) in order to reduce the risk.

Rough drying

Rough drying is, quite simply, drying your hair with a hairdryer in a rough manner. Rough drying in a salon environment typically refers to a quick blast with a hairdryer in a carefree manner, with the sole aim of drying the hair, irrespective of how it looks. For straight-haired people this can be a way of drying that results in a perfectly wearable look. For curly-haired people it is mostly going to be the absolute worst possible way to dry your hair.

✱ If you have the hair for it
If you have the type of curly hair that can take rough drying, you are a rare exception among curly folk. Certain curl types can take it – only fortunate curly-haired people with a curl pattern that is so perfectly formed into ringlets that their curls' structure can endure being blasted. When drying this curl type in such a rough manner, I would still hold the dryer further from the hair and definitely use it without the nozzle attached. The nozzle increases the pressure from the dryer and is likely to cause a certain amount of frizz in even the hardiest of curls. At a guess, I would say I encounter this type of curl shape in less than one in 100 people. You probably know if this is you, because you have most likely been drying your hair like this for years. Consider yourself lucky.

✱ If you don't really have the hair for it, but are either lazy or time-starved
Rough drying can still be a styling option for other curl types, but expect to apply a greater degree of effort to finish it nicely and with a less curly result. For looser curl types or wavy hair, rough drying can result in straight hair. If your hair straightens simply by being roughly blasted, I would consider straight to be a much less damaging way to wear your hair. If you have a more intense curl, you can still try drying your hair this way, but allow for a frighteningly fluffy or frizzy moment between it being dry and being a wearable look. Start with wet hair and use a hairdryer without the nozzle. You can experiment with leaving some conditioner in or applying a styling product at this stage, but you will almost certainly be using product once dry, so don't use too much when wet. Gently dry your hair consistently throughout until it is fully dry. If you wish, you can brush your hair carefully with a soft brush, being sure to brush the ends then the mid-lengths and finally from root to tip. End by raking your fingers through your hair, adding a serum or defining cream as you go. Depending on your hair type you will find your hair either has a wonderful beachy wave, or – if it isn't suited to this method – is a total mess. Do experiment: it could turn out to be the key that unlocks another way to wear your hair.

'Plopping'

At Unruly Curls we like to use as little heat as possible to style hair and sometimes use the American trend of hair 'plopping'. We have found that it works better for people with thicker hair rather than those with finer hair. With the latter, you have to be really careful not to pull the curls out at the hairline.

You can use a pin or a hair tie to secure it in place à la Princess Leia.

1. Spread a cloth or towel down on a flat surface, then lean over it and place your head against the surface, positioning the hair onto it so that all the curls are concentrated on the top of the head.

2. Put the far edge of the cloth over your head at the nape of the neck. Grab the sides of the cloth and start twisting them away from your face. It should look like two big twists on the sides of your head.

3. Once you feel that the rolls are tight enough, straighten your body out and twist the rolls towards the back of your head in a bun. You can use a pin or a hair tie to secure it in place à la Princess Leia.

4. Leave it on for as long as you wish; usually about 20 minutes is enough for hair to dry.

5. After you remove the plop, make sure you don't touch the curls while they're still wet so they keep the definition and don't frizz.

47

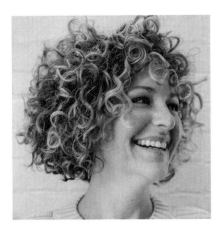

The dreaded 'Day Two'

This is probably the section I expect most curly-haired people to flip to when picking up this book. It is by far the topic I am most frequently quizzed on.

Over the years I have explored just about every conceivable solution to make day two anything other than a 'scraped-back-in-a-bun' day. My earlier, pathetic answers were mostly bonkers ideas like sleeping facedown with a snorkel to breathe through, sleeping upright in an armchair, not sleeping, living your life only in day one by washing on a daily basis, and all kinds of other junk ideas. After years of peddling such random nonsense, I started to accept that I needed to think a bit harder in order to help people overcome the challenge of the dreaded day two.

Ultimately, making 'day one' curls look amazing will promote much higher odds of 'day two' looking passable. I strongly encourage my clients to invest the time it takes to get their curls looking as good as they can on the day they wash them, factoring in that after sleeping on them, the hair will undoubtedly suffer to a certain extent and be less defined. The nature of curly hair is that contact of any kind is generally unwelcome for well-defined curls and likely to be the cause of frizz. Beyond going for gold on day one, the following tips will surely help.

PINEAPPLE OR TOPKNOT WHEN SLEEPING

This seems obvious, but somehow escapes many as a solution to day two hair. Carefully, without applying too much tension, gather your hair into a loose topknot. This should maintain the definition of much of your hair, possibly resulting in only the undersides of your hair being unsettled by a night's sleep. Be sure not to pull your hair too straight when putting it into a topknot. The heat and pressure of your head on the pillow will result in a lasting straightening effect when you wake. Try using a hair bungee (see page 81), which won't meddle with your tresses, instead of potentially messing up your curls with a hairband.

SILK OR SATIN PILLOWCASE This is an old-school beauty tip that was apparently a favourite of Max Factor back in the 50s, and it truly helps curls to stay intact throughout the night. Silk pillowcases were promoted as a beauty tip, because they were believed to prevent wrinkles. Replacing a cotton pillowcase with a much finer, smoother satin or, even better, silk pillowcase, will result in a noticeable reduction in the amount of frizz caused when sleeping. Cotton may feel soft to the touch, but for our hair the fibres can be highly unsettling. The natural fibres of silk are also believed to moderate temperature, helping us stay cool when we are hot and warm when we are cold. I suggest this simple step to almost all of my clients. So far I have only had positive reports of how much it helps curly hair stay defined. Well worth a try. If it's good enough for Marilyn, it's good enough for me...

RE-WETTING YOUR HAIR IN THE MORNING ON DAY TWO This is what I imagine most people attempt when waking to messed up bed-head curls. It can be done in many ways. When I quiz my clients on how they do this, I am often alarmed to find they have gone about it in totally the wrong way. The right way is to start by shaking your head upside down. Using a spray bottle of water with the nozzle set to create a fine mist, rather than a spurt of water, mist water through the ends and mid-lengths of your hair, avoiding the roots and being careful not to totally drench your hair. Soak your hands with water and apply a small amount of defining cream between your palms and fingers. Keep your fingers together, creating paddles out of your hands to avoid tugging and picking or combing your hair with separated fingers. Scrunch and swipe past your hair, taking care not to pull at it.

Using wet hands will allow the product to impart onto your damp hair without disturbing it. Having damp or dry hair and dry hands covered in a sticky product will usually cause more of a disturbance than having wet hands. The action is one of glancing your hands over your curls to smooth whatever frizziness might have occurred during sleep.

When scrunching, be sure to remove your hands from your hair via the exact same path they entered by. Be extra careful not to snag, drag, pick or comb your curls. The technique to perfect is one of compacting by scrunching and lightly glancing against your hair, ensuring that you are not separating or flattening your curls. You can then either allow your hair to dry naturally or use a diffuser.

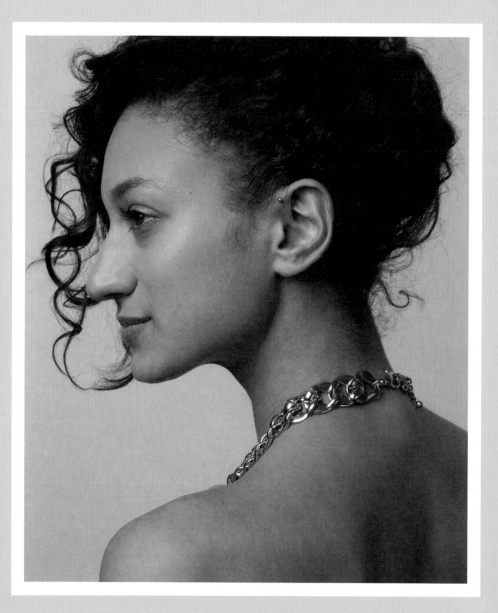

Up dos

Curly hair is perfectly suited to up dos: half the work is already done. It is easy when you have an understanding of the key basics and the confidence to try it out. I am frequently asked what can be done to achieve different up-styles and rarely does anyone seem confident enough to even give it a go. It's totally worth taking a bit of time to learn; up-styles provide an excellent alternative look to your norm and can totally make an outfit or look.

PREPARATION Preparation is EVERYTHING when starting an up-style. It is crucial to all up dos. Expecting freshly washed, conditioned and dried hair to stay in place is wildly unrealistic. Hair is most likely to be easiest to wear up when it is either slightly dirty or with a decent amount of tack to it. This can be achieved with hairspray or almost any product. Don't overdo it but make sure your hair has something in it to help it grip.

FOUNDATION Creating a foundation to the style is another essential step to ensuring a lasting do. Look at any up do and consider that at the heart of it probably exists a firmly placed secure point, to which the whole look is attached.

BASIC UP DO HOW-TOS The most basic way to start is to determine the area that the hair will be piled onto or dressed around. Take a small section, enough to secure into a small ponytail.

Up dos are the perfect style for 'Day Two' hair

Ideally, do not include hair from the hairline. If you have thick hair you can take a smaller section, and with finer hair you might need to take a larger section. The area drawn into the band that is stretched flat against the scalp will become the anchor to which you can loosely pin all the other sections. Simply take the hanging sections that are not in the banded ponytail, position them with your finger wherever you desire, and pin them to the flat, secured area. Gradually pick up all the hair, section by section or curl by curl, and when all the free-hanging curls are in place, grab the ponytail section that hangs from the centre and gather it on top of itself, and pin that into place too. For a high quiff style, place the secure banded section forward of the top of the head. If the style is to accentuate an asymmetric dress, try positioning the small ponytail section to one side of the nape of the neck. If you look at any curly up-style, the vast majority can be created using this technique. Most importantly, this approach ensures that the whole style is as secure as the small ponytail at its core.

51

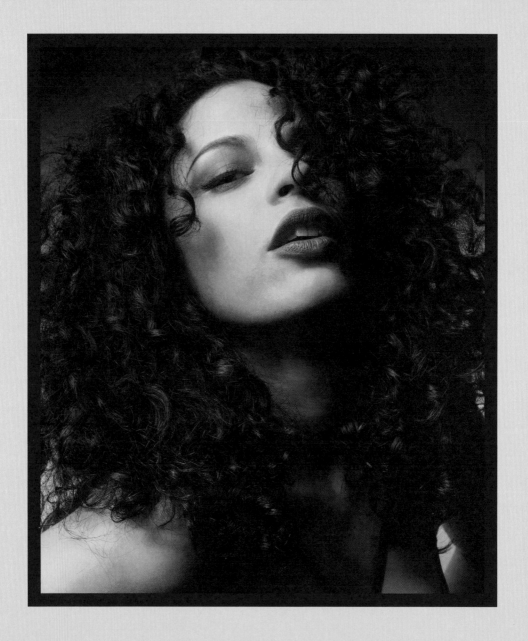

CURL CASE: RUAMA

ETHNICITY: BRAZILIAN

Brazil is a country of diversity: Indigenous, Europeans, Africans and Asians; we are all mixed. Brazilians are now in a proud hair revolution: our curls are now trendy.

My hair always had waves but when I hit puberty, to my mother's desperation, my waves turned into small curls. I wasn't able to tie my own hair up to go to school, so my mother cut my hair like a boy! From that point on my life's goal was to make my hair grow again, and I decided to use chemical straightener. We called it a Japanese blowdry, and I started this when I was 14. I needed to use chemicals every week and straighten the roots every four months. 14 years later, I left my hometown where I was a TV presenter (let's just say straight hair was considered a more commercial look) to live in Sao Paulo, a huge, modern, cosmopolitan city, so I could let my hair grow free of chemicals. I met my real hair again.

Coming to London, it was a surprise to see how people here love 'Brazilian hair', even selling it as extensions. Now I really can feel amazing with my naturally curly, voluminous Brazilian hair.

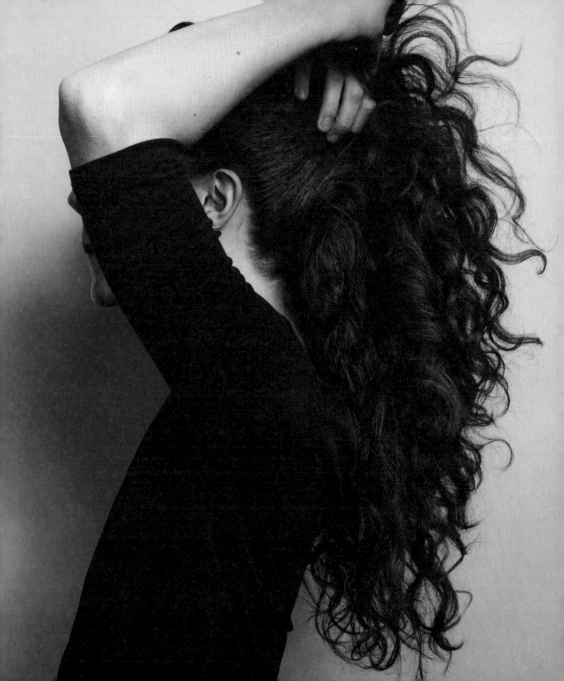

Great hair starts with a great cut. Find out how to pick the best hairdressers, avoid the bad ones, and ask for what you need.

Cutting Curly Hair

CHAPTER 4

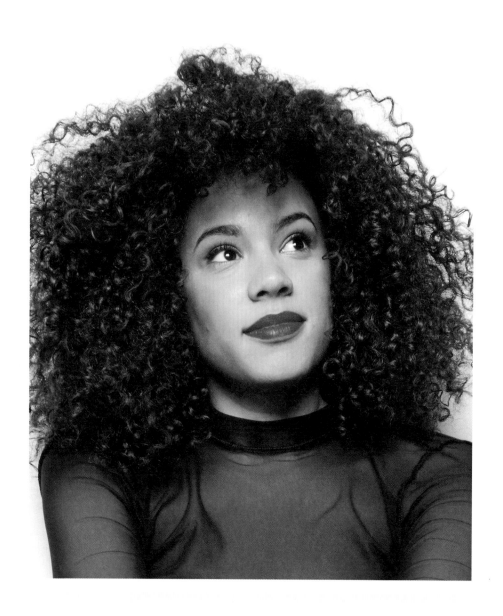

The perfect cut

The best haircuts work with the hair, rather than against it. As always, embrace your curls – don't fight them.

How to cut curly hair

Cutting curly hair becomes less difficult when a hairdresser has a good understanding of how to utilise layering and the shrinking capacity of hair after even a small amount of weight has been removed. Finding a hairdresser that understands how vital it is to see a client's hair dry as near to naturally as is possible in the course of a haircut appointment, instead of just impressing on you how sleek and orderly it looks when dried into a nice style that is just hiding a bad haircut, is a good start. A hairdresser who understands curly hair will work with hair dried in a natural way. Cutting until a good shape is achieved is part of being able to cut curly hair well.

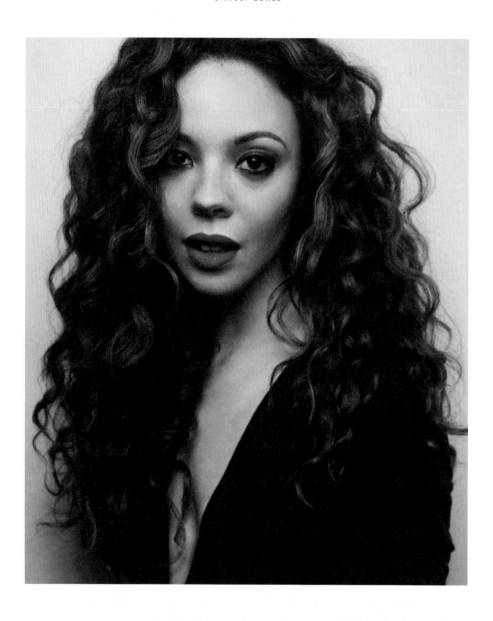

How to find a stylist and avoid a bad cut

Seek out the best, ditch the rest.

✱ **DO your research.** The internet is a valuable resource.

✱ **DO stop and ask curly-haired people** in your area where they get their hair cared for and if they would recommend anyone in particular.

✱ **DO book in for a wash and dry and consultation.** If they can't dry your hair nicely with its natural texture, they likely won't be able to cut it nicely either.

✱ **DO arrive with your hair dried naturally,** so that your stylist can see its natural texture.

✱ **DO take along photos of styles you like** – it really helps. Try to find photos of hair that has a similar texture to yours.

✱ **DO ask who is the salon's busiest stylist,** or who is the most difficult to get an appointment with. This will usually put you in the chair of someone who is in demand and has some skills.

✱ **DO NOT go in asking for a radical transformation on your first visit.** Let the hairdresser prove him- or herself by simply giving your hair a trim first.

✱ **DO NOT tell them what you want straight away.** Save that for after they have been given a chance to tell you what they think you ought to do with your curls.

✱ **DO NOT go through with the appointment** if you sense the stylist is uneasy or seems intimidated. If your stylist is stressed, you will be too.

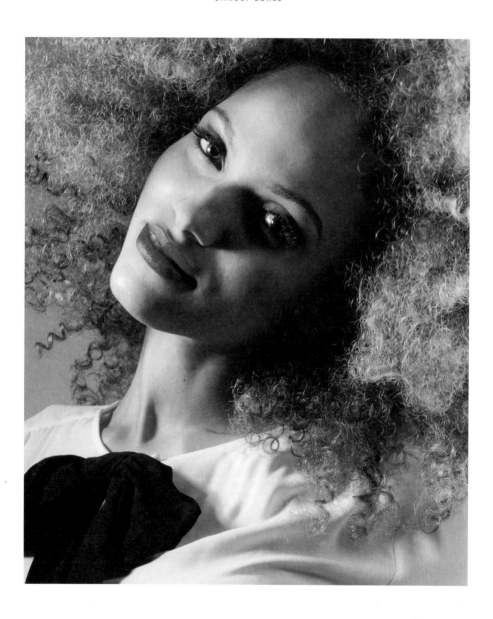

Choosing a style to suit you

Your hairstyle should be as unique as you are.

Every beauty editor, beauty blogger, journalist and columnist, everywhere, bangs on about how important it is to find a hairstyle that suits your face shape. Hairdressers promote it as one of the main skills in their profession, which defines them and sets them apart in their ability. Choosing a hairstyle to suit a particular face shape is far from a one-size-fits-all approach, so it's key to find a stylist who understands this.

It's not just the shape of your face that needs to be taken into account, it's your body shape as well. Everything has to be in balance! If you are transitioning from highly groomed, sleek hair back to your natural curls, your stylist will have to take this into account. They should also consider other aspects individual to you, such as your personal style and whether you wear glasses. Assessing a client's style options and their candidacy for a new shape is an essential part of the initial consultation so be sure to ask for this and allow extra time if necessary. A good hairdresser will expect this and welcome it. Don't settle for less!

Cutting methods

————————

Each method has its place, and it's key to find a hairdresser who knows the difference.

WET CUT Throughout a conventional wet cut, the stylist may be able to assess the length and shape it will have when dry. The client, however, will have little or no idea regarding the length and the shape the cut will sit in until it has been completely dried curly in the way they would normally wear it (something that is difficult to recreate on the day if the client normally wears their hair dried naturally). It can be harrowing for a client to see their hair being pulled straight and then cut. It is essential for the stylist to evaluate the different areas of the scalp and the nature of the hair growing from the various parts (see Growth patterns and partings on page 45) in order to prevent a huge disconnect between areas where the hair is more tightly wound and other areas where it falls in a looser pattern.

DRY CUT Dry cutting can be done in several ways but, for the most part, it refers to the method of curl-by-curl cutting: identifying a curl, picking it up and cutting it, then moving on to the next curl. It takes a great deal of confidence and experience to master this technique, and isn't as easy as it looks.

With dry cutting, a hairdresser can more accurately detect areas of damage, as well as differences in the frequency of the curl pattern. For the client, this also affords the opportunity to see how the cut is evolving. In my view, this more 'organic' hands-on approach is excellent, especially if a client arrives with naturally dried curls, so it's possible to see how the hair falls naturally.

However, there are occasions when this doesn't work so well. If the hair has been tied, pinned or clipped up at any point since it was last washed, for example, some areas will be straighter than normal. If hair condition is poor and there are lots of split ends, the risk of missing these is higher with a dry cut, and the condition of the hair can deteriorate more rapidly than might be expected.

This method also relies on curl clusters forming in the same way each time the hair is washed and dried. With experience I can say that this is not the case. My preference will always be to evaluate a client's suitability for either method. Most frequently I opt

62

Arrive at the salon with hair that has dried naturally

for a combination of the two methods. Sometimes I draft the basic shape dry in a freehand style, then wet it and retrace the outline of the provisional draft, to ensure that all of the ends are cut in a balanced and controlled way, then dry it curly.

RAZOR CUTTING AND THINNING The idea of asking your hairdresser to thin out your thick, curly hair has an obvious appeal. Many hairdressers even suggest it and see it as a suitable method of reducing the overall mass of hair, making it easier to manage and quicker to dry. While this initially seems to make a great deal of sense, there are drawbacks.

The shape of a single strand of curly hair is affected by its length, so creating various lengths throughout a section or cluster of hair by razor cutting or using thinning scissors can be problematic. In a cluster of curls you will have a mix of new hair growing and a certain amount of broken hairs. These shorter hairs dry tighter than the longer ones, with the latter hanging looser under their own weight. The shorter hairs separate and the ends stick out, distorting the cluster's sleekness and making it appear frizzier. Thinning or razor cutting has a tendency to increase the occurrence of frizz.

Perhaps an even greater issue I have with cutting techniques that venture too far into the interior of

the hair is that the shorter hairs become inaccessible. No hairdresser, no matter how skilled or motivated, will ever be able to retrace their exact footsteps through a previous haircut that used thinning scissors. So, once thinned, the shorter hairs will have to wait for as long as it takes to grow out to the same length as the rest of the hair before being cut again. For this reason, I advise my clients to turn to other techniques to make their hair feel manageable.

LAYERING The cut most feared by curly-haired people is the Triangle. Most people with curly hair have suffered a version of it and its just plain awful. So how do you avoid the dreaded Triangle? By layering your hair. Watch out, because with too many layers you can end up like Louis XIV or Charles II. Not enough and you can exaggerate the Triangle by adding enough volume to add further width but not enough to get lift at the crown. Well-executed layers are essential for curly hair.

MAINTENANCE CUTS It is really common for curly-haired people to go for a long time between cuts, likely due to the fear of exposure to another bad haircut. I typically recommend 3–4 months between cuts. However, shorter styles and hair that is in poorer condition need more frequent trimming. If you are trying to grow your hair, I definitely suggest regular haircuts to keep your hair healthy.

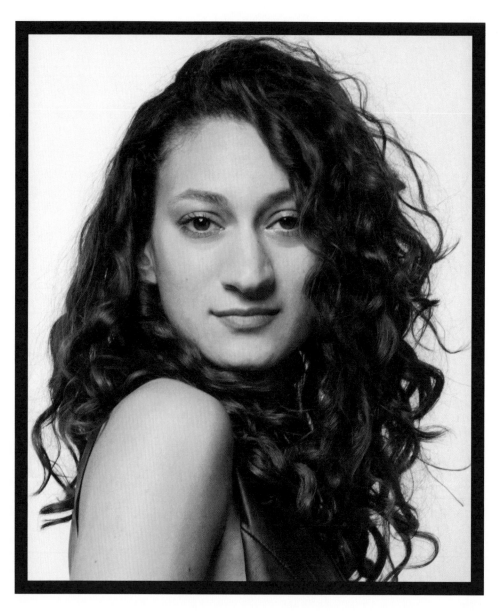

CURL CASE: NICOLA

ETHNICITY: MEDITERRANEAN

My Mediterranean roots spring through my hair in tight coils and loose curls that have never been easy to tame. As a child, I always wore the mop look well and it took a while for my hair to grow beyond my shoulders before my curls conceded to gravity. Even then, it was near impossible to comb my hair and so I often had it in plaits.

Curly hair doesn't come with a user's manual, so I spent much of my teenage years experimenting with care routines and hair products. When my curls were tighter I used leave-in conditioner to avoid dryness and damage. However, it never held my hair for long and would frizz out soon after I washed it. I resorted to using styling mousse but that seemed to cement my curls in place.

Once I found the right hairdresser and products I began loving the process of styling my hair. I learnt how to diffuse it properly in order to work the curls. I now love having it down: it's my best accessory.

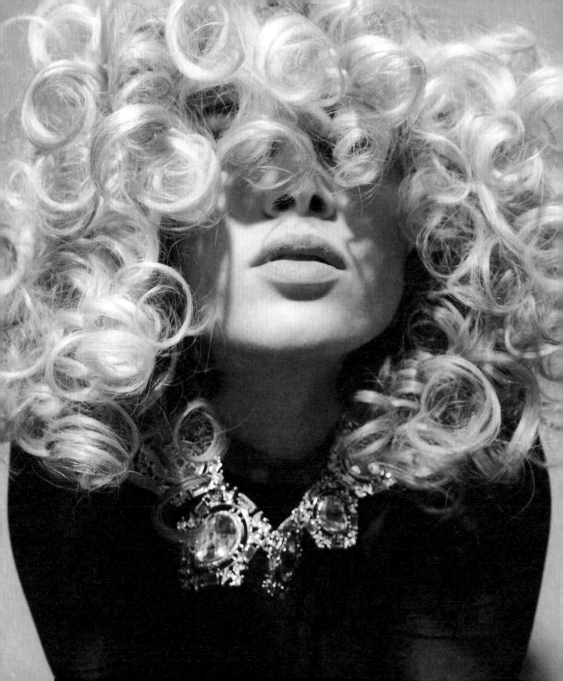

Blonde, brunette or rainbow-haired... no matter
the colour you choose, you need to do it right.

Colouring Curly Hair

CHAPTER 5

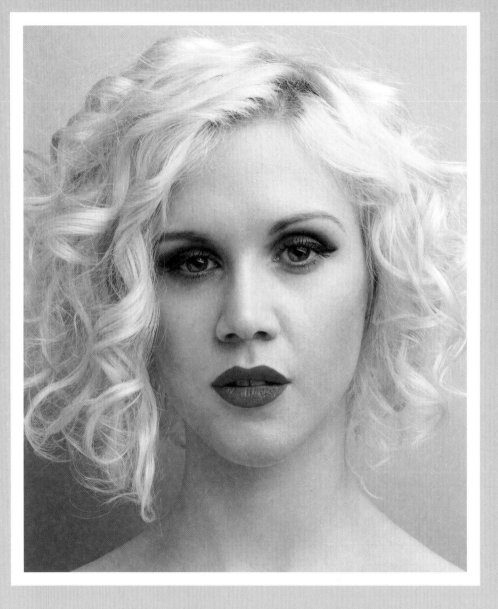

Colouring care and maintenance

———

It's possible to make your curls darker, lighter or even neon bright, as long as you do it properly and take care whenever you need to expose your hair to harsh chemicals.

69

Avoiding damage

———

Chemicals and bleach pose a risk of damage to any hair, but curly-haired people need to be particularly careful as our hair is prone to dryness and breakage. Curly hair reflects light easily, so when it comes to colour, less is more.

The key to avoiding damage is to keep the moisture content of the hair as high as possible before colouring. Prevention is better than cure, so make sure you follow the tips in the Curl Care chapter (pages 25–37) to build a strong foundation.

PRE-COLOUR Wash your hair before going into the salon when having your hair coloured. I would encourage you to use natural oils a week before you come in for your appointment, but make sure these are totally washed out before you come in because oil coats the hair, which makes it difficult for colour to take.

POST-COLOUR Ideally, wait at least three days to wash your hair after having it coloured. If you can hold out for slightly longer – say, a week – I would definitely recommend it. It can take a minumum of three days for the hair cuticle layer to close and trap the colour molecule, so wait for as long as you can.

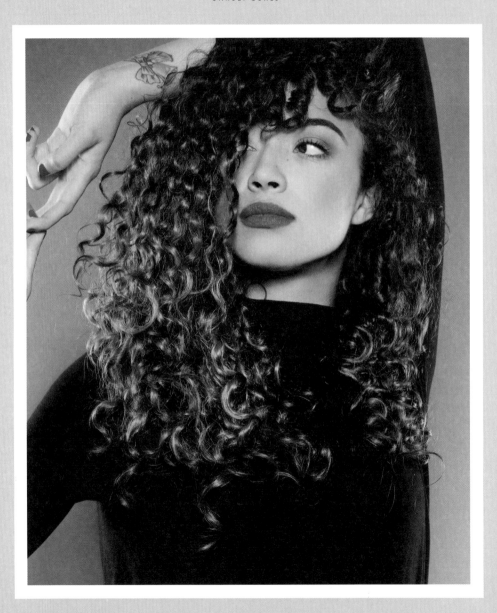

Colouring products

The best products are those that colour the hair without being too harsh. Generally, staying the same shade or darker will be less damaging and going lighter will almost certainly do damage.

L'Oreal and Wella do excellent high-lift tints which offer up to four shades lighter without bleach, so you avoid the dreaded straw-like and straightening effect of overbleached crispy strands. Basically any products that are used professionally, properly and minimally will limit the damage inherent with colouring.

Home colouring is generally better done when you have consulted a hair colourist: the history of colour on your hair and its condition should be assessed by a professional so that they can advise you which type to use. I am a big fan of Herbatint permanent dyes. They are organic products that are suitable for vegans, offering excellent grey coverage and with around 30 shades to choose from. However, they are not able to lighten your hair, only offering the same shade or darker coverage.

When colouring your hair, use a deep conditioner such as Shea Moisture Jamaican Black Castor Oil Strengthen & Restore Treatment Masque (see page 111) but do not use deep conditioners in the days before colouring, as they will interfere with the functioning of almost any hair colourant.

Prevention is always better than cure

Maintenance

Curly-haired people shouldn't shampoo too often anyway (see page 30), but this is especially true if you colour your hair. Leave it as long as possible between washes, or co-wash (see page 28). This will help to stop your colour from fading too quickly.

It's now become something of a trend to have visible roots, but if you don't like this look your curly hair will give you an advantage, as the added volume will mean any regrowth takes longer to become visible. You can cover regrowth of grey hairs temporarily with root mascara or powder pens.

With lighter colours, be careful not to overdo it. Consider all lightening colours as damaging; therefore, the less you have the better. Blonde colour can be very addictive though: the more you have, the more you need to have!

71

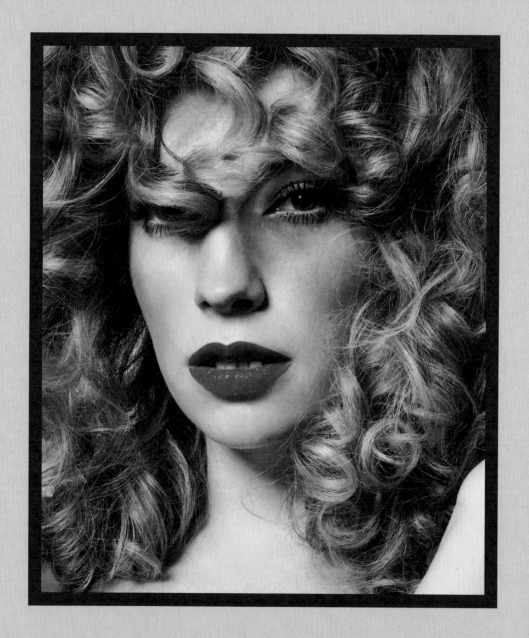

CURL CASE: GRACE

ETHNICITY: ENGLISH

If I could go back in time, I would definitely tell my
16-year-old self not to straighten
my natural curls.

I straightened my hair all throughout secondary school
until I went on a two-week holiday to Turkey and forgot
my straighteners. I got so many compliments on my big
hair, I've kept it natural ever since!

Now I love my big curly hair: it defines me and makes me
feel unique. I would tell anyone with natural curls to do
the same.

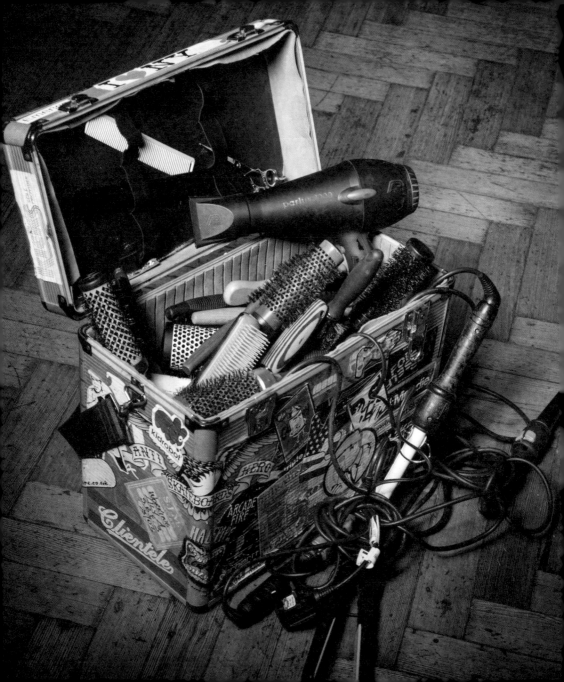

When you've got a thick, curly mane, it's essential
to have the proper tools for the job — they will
work wonders for your hair.

The Toolkit

CHAPTER 6

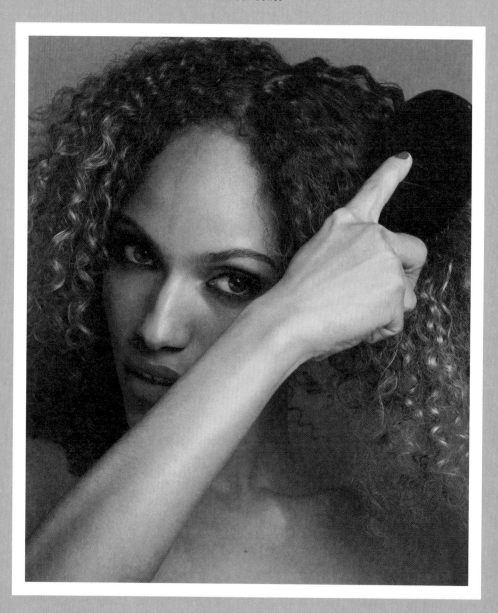

The right tools for the job

You need decent tools to care and style your curly hair – those which protect and enhance your beautiful locks.

Often, I hear my clients say that they can never get their hair to look the way I do once I have styled it in the salon. Fair enough – I guess I am the expert. Or is it simply that I have the right tools for the job?

Years ago, I was at a friend's house before a night out and she asked if I would dry her hair. No problem – until she handed me her pathetic hairdryer. I was rendered unable to do even a half-decent job and thus realised a big problem: a lot of people are working with terrible tools.

Most people buy their tools on the high street, whereas no hairdresser would go anywhere near these products as they know the advantages of a proper hair and beauty supply shop. Avoid the cheap tools and always look for nice finishing; rough edges and poorly finished plastics can wreck hair.

Keep your tools clean and free of hair. Take care not to wrap the flex of powered tools around the tool itself to avoid damaging the wire, and always make sure you have the right tool for the job – the wrong one will almost certainly fail you.

The toolkit

BRUSHES

There is a right and wrong brush for every purpose.

Using the wrong brush in the wrong way can be very bad for your hair. You must be extra careful to select the right kind. The brush I most commonly use for detangling curly hair before washing is a vanity brush, sometimes called a grooming brush.

These brushes are the most effective at detangling dry curly hair without harming it. They have a mixture of natural black/brown boar bristles and white nylon bristles. The fact that the bristles are set into a cushioned pad allows them to flex when tension is applied. This feature makes them particularly suitable for curly hair, because they release the hair, rather than snapping it, when too forcefully or aggressively applied. The nylon bristles detangle the hair, and the shorter natural boar bristles draw natural oils from the root down the shaft. As with combing, it is important to start by brushing the tips or ends of your hair. The most popular brand of this brush is Mason Pearson. They are expensive, hand-made in the UK, and well worth every penny. However, there is a much cheaper variant of this type of brush made by Denman, which is also perfectly good too. They come in three sizes.

After washing, you can brush through hair when wet to get out any large tangles. I like to use the Tangle Teezer hairbrushes as the way the teeth are arranged means that they do not pull the hair so much. It is best to avoid brushing hair when dry and ready to style as this can cause frizz – use a comb instead.

COMBS

Look for combs that are finished nicely with no sharp edges on any surfaces that will be in direct contact with your hair.

Avoid plastic combs completely – they will generate static and frizz, and can lead to hair breakage. Go for a wooden comb, or better still, get an anti-static or carbon one, all of which will generate less static. Make sure the comb has wide enough teeth to do the job efficiently, and not so fine that they cause lots of resistance and end up pulling and stretching wet hair as you work through it.

Comb through hair in gentle strokes, first combing the ends of the hair and gradually working upwards to ease out any tangles. Slow and steady wins the race.

STRAIGHTENING IRONS

Straightening irons come in many variations, with plates of different sizes coated in different substances, from ceramic or tourmaline, to provide as flat and smooth a surface as possible. Be warned – it is very rare for manufacturers to publicise the actual temperatures of their irons.

Some irons have curved edges to their plates and it is suggested that this feature can be used to create curls or waves. This way of styling is one of the worst things you can do to curly hair. It works on hair the same way that paper curls when being pulled around the edge of a ruler. Stretching hair while heating to such a high temperature is most definitely going to result in severe damage quite quickly.
Don't do it!

DRYERS

**Of all the tools a curly-haired person needs to get right,
the most important is their hairdryer.**

My preferred way to dry curly hair is and always will be to dry it naturally without a dryer. However, in today's busy, modern world the hairdryer is usually relied upon to ensure a speedy drying time.

There are two main components to a hairdryer. The most important is the motor, which produces and delivers the flow of air. The second is the heat element. The heat element turns the air into hot air. A good hairdryer will typically have a more powerful motor and a less aggressive heat element, drying hair by moving a greater volume of moderately-heated air through the hair. Expensive dryers will often feature the added benefit of a switch to select a lower heat.

Do not be fooled by the word 'professional' being pasted along the side of a hairdryer, but choose one where the motor is rated at or above 1800 watts to ensure a powerful device. Ensure that is has selectable heat settings. A hairdryer that has a standardised aperture at the nozzle end is convenient when buying additional aftermarket 'universal fit' accessories, such as diffusers and pick nozzles.

My preferred hairdryer is a Parlux Superturbo 3000 with a matte black finish. It has a really long flex and is virtually indestructible. I dry about 10 heads of curls a day, five days a week, and my Parlux lasts for several years. The matte coating provides excellent grip in wet hands.

DIFFUSERS AND HOT-SOCKS

The diffuser works by literally diffusing the flow of air from the hairdryer.

The direct flow of hot air from the dryer is buffeted around in a small space within the diffuser, and the small holes allow the hot air to flow from a broader area, with a substantially decreased air pressure. Without a diffuser the flow of air, even on a low setting, will straighten curly hair and distort the curl, leaving it undefined and frizzy.

Hot socks are a fantastic invention consisting of a mesh fabric with an elasticated opening that fits around the end of any dryer. They perform the same function as other diffusers and provide an excellent solution for travelling light. Just pack them with the rest of your socks!

ACCESSORIES

Curly hair can snag easily, so look for well-made accessories.

Avoid clips and ornamental accessories with rough edges, especially those with metal hinged parts, as they can damage hair by getting caught. Regular hairbands are okay but hair bungees are best – lengths of elastic that have small hooks at each end and allow you to determine the exact tautness of your ponytail. Wear it looser while less active to give your hair a break from being stretched and crimped. The real advantage of bungees over regular hairbands is that they do not require pulling your curly ponytail through an increasingly smaller elastic which will disturb your defined curls each time. They also offer control over the tautness, unlike regular elastics.

81

CURLING TONGS

Much in the same way as straightening irons are likely to cause damage, curling tongs are capable of drying out your hair and can have a negative impact on your hair's health.

If you do use curling tongs, I would strongly encourage you to look for a set that features selectable heat dials or switches. Try to use your tongs on the lowest setting possible and be sure not to over-expose your hair by holding it in them for only a few seconds. Any sort of heat only causes damage.

In the same way that twisting curls randomly can cause damage when done without regard for the natural direction the curls flows in, when selecting a section of hair to be tonged I recommend bobbing it in your palm to identify its natural direction, then winding it around the tong in the same direction.

Ensure that the ends of your hair are neatly wrapped around the barrel of the tong and turn it, wrapping the extended hair around the barrel as it winds toward the root.

Hold your section of hair in place for several seconds before releasing it. Be sure to allow the freshly curled section to cool before touching: it is the cooling process that will ensure the curl lasts.

One thing to remember is that the bigger the section of hair and barrel of the tong, the looser the curl will be. The smaller the section of hair and barrel of the tong, the tighter the curl will be.

CURL STYLERS

These tools are a relatively recent invention. They create perfect curls by drawing a section of hair through a mechanism that simultaneously heats and forges a spiral shape into the hair.

Be aware that these automated tools are unable to identify the natural path of the hair's curl pattern and, as a result, they are likely to force many of the curls against their natural pattern, while at the same time heating them. This process is the most damaging to your hair's health and physical structure.

My recommendation is to avoid this kind of tool. If you must use them, make sure your hair is properly hydrated and use a heat protection spray.

HEATED ROLLERS

Heated rollers are by far the least damaging heated tool you can use, due to them reaching a temperature that is perfectly tolerable for curly hair.

When used properly, they are very effective at changing tight curls into looser waves and they are fantastic at creating volume at the root.

Unfortunately, most people find them not only difficult to use but also relatively ineffective compared to heated curling tongs. You need to roll and secure them tightly into damp or nearly dry hair and keep them in the hair until it is completely dry for them to have the desired result. It's worth it, though, to achieve those beautifully bouncy waves without damaging your hair.

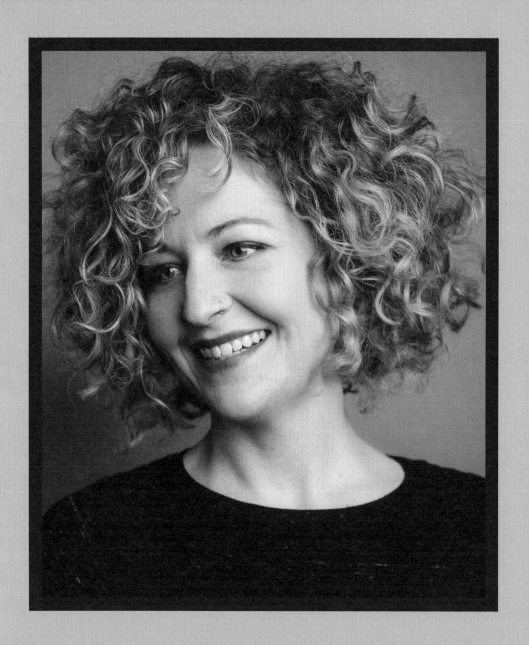

CURL CASE: HERMIONE

ETHNICITY: BRITISH/IRISH

I was born bald and stayed that way until I was about 18 months old, when seemingly out of nowhere sprung a head of tight, strawberry blonde curls. Adorable, right? Not so much when it came to brushing my hair, which turned into a daily battle between me and my mum.

Being the only one in my immediately family with curly hair, no one really knew what to do with it. Ditto for hairdressers. My biggest disappointment hit after a haircut when I was 13 where I asked to look like Rachel from *Friends* but after one blowdry at home, looked more like Simba from *The Lion King*.

I floated through my teenage years with a slight curl revival – this included heavy use of hair mousse and no diffuser in sight. I just accepted that my hair would be frizzy so turned to straightening irons most of the time.

Finding a stylist who knows and understands the hair they're working with has made such a difference! I use fewer products, wash my hair less and have totally embraced my curls. It's been almost 10 years since I've used straighteners and I will never look back.

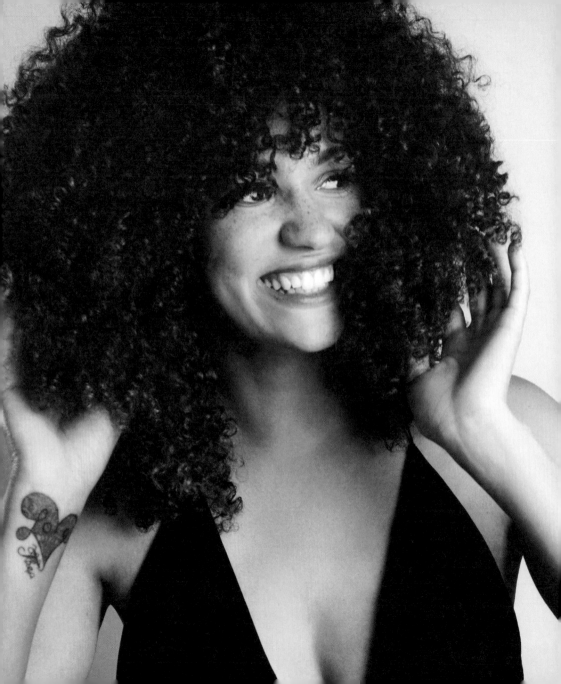

There are certain situations and hair types that require some extra TLC.

Special Care Hair

CHAPTER 7

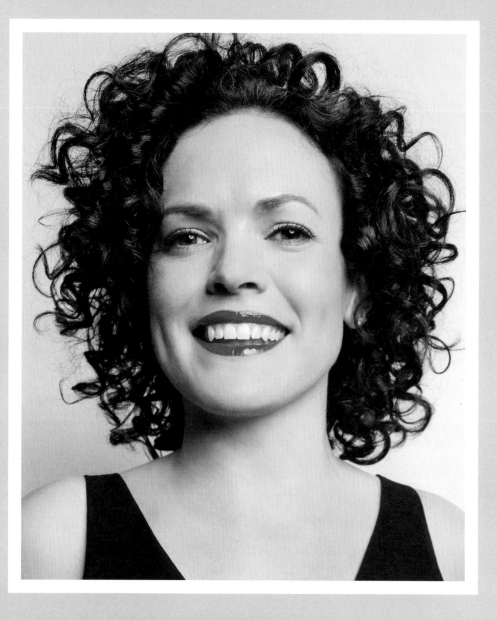

Myth busters

There are so many myths surrounding curly hair that a book could be written on these alone!

✱ **MYTH: Curls never grow long**
✱ **FACT:** All hair types are capable of growing, but it does take a little more time and patience for curly hair. One reason is that growth isn't always as noticeable because of the shrinkage of the curl. This is all dependent on the health of your hair, which is partly determined by your genes, but also by external factors. Check out pages 28–29 for tips on keeping your hair as healthy as possible.

✱ **MYTH: Brushing curly hair regularly can lead to straighter tresses**
✱ **FACT:** Brushing naturally curly hair agitates the curls, causing a frizzy look which we all try to avoid, but these straighter looking, stretched out curls won't last for long. Also, brushing can lead to breakage, so you need to be careful. Use your fingers to loosen the curls instead of a brush. And make sure only to do it when your hair is damp.

✱ **MYTH: Curls aren't professional**
✱ **FACT:** There's an idea that curly hair isn't for the office, particularly in less creative industries. But we say that well-groomed, beautifully maintained curls are acceptable anywhere – and we're not alone. So make sure your hair is the best version of itself and conquer your work environment with confidence.

✱ **MYTH: Regular washing will dry up curly hair**
✱ **FACT:** If you have a tendency towards a greasy scalp, then regular washing is actually good for curly hair. We are fans of the co-washing ethos (see page 28); however, different scalps mean different hair care regimes and if you use lots of product on your hair then you are likely to have greater build-up and grime, which needs to be washed away. If you don't, it can actually weaken the hair follicles and make them greasy.

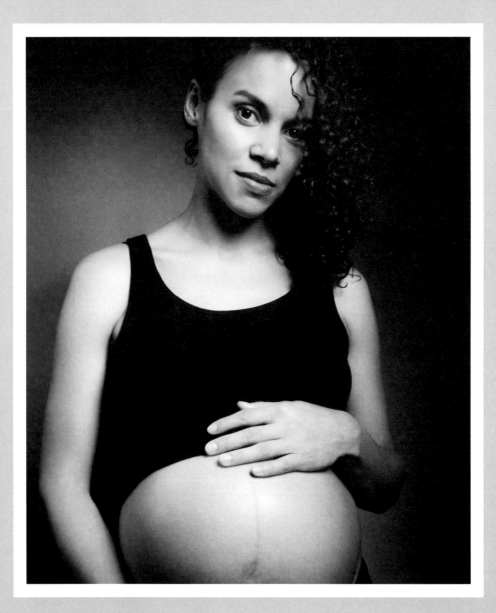

Pregnancy

———

Pregnancy can cause drastic changes to the hair.

Hair follicles are very delicate and can be affected by a number of things including puberty, pregnancy or menopause. For example, you may find that your once wavy hair becomes a bountiful head of ringlets. However, the hair will usually return to its former type and texture in time. But managing your new hair may be a completely foreign experience.

During pregnancy, increased hormone levels bring changes to your hair – often making it more luxurious and abundant as you 'bloom'. But after birth, levels return to normal. There is often some initial hair loss but hormones stabilise and normal hair cycles will return, usually after about three months.

HOW TO CARE FOR HAIR AFTER PREGNANCY
Use ultra-delicate and natural products that encourage hair replenishment and growth. Often, brands specially formulated for babies are mild enough for you to use during this time.

At each stage of your post-birth recovery, your hair will grow in different thicknesses. Getting your hair trimmed every six weeks will make sure your hair is always growing at its thickest and best, as well as giving you a much-needed treat.

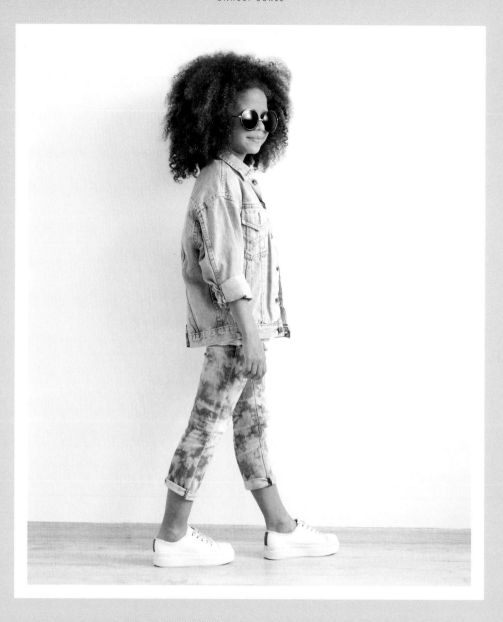

Kids

Helping your child to get a handle on their curls as early as possible will set them up for a stress-free curly life.

Bath time, like bed time, is a hassle for kids even if as adults they become things we enjoy. With the right approach from as early as possible a curly-haired child can master control of their curls for life.

Taking a child to the salon is a potentially traumatic experience for all involved. Try to find one that is welcoming to children. Take along plenty to occupy them and don't get too excited about it. Ideally, sit them on your lap and try to find a hairdresser that will take the time to familiarise themselves with some friendly chatter prior to whipping out the shears.

As with all curly hair, get it cut frequently. Children's hair is just as likely, if not more likely, to get tangled and roughed up. Having healthy, well-cared-for and frequently trimmed hair will save a lot of stress down the line.

If you make sure you have enough time, patience and the right products and tools, your child will grow to love and care for their curls as much as you do.

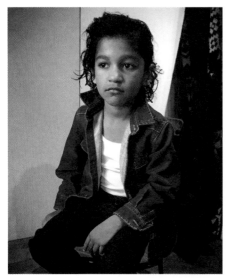
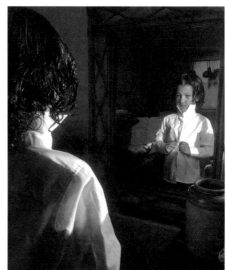
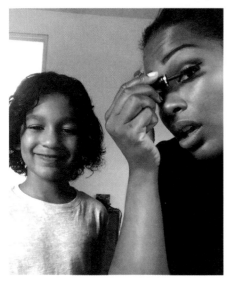
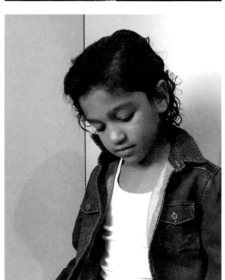

CURL CASE: ROMAN

ETHNICITY: JAMAICAN/INDIAN & ENGLISH/ITALIAN
MUM: SHARMADEAN

Before I had Roman, I would always see mixed race kids with mums who couldn't do their hair. It took me back to how my mum did my hair – it was really painful.

I did some research and found that conditioner was a key element that hadn't been present in my childhood. I got into a routine where I would gently brush his hair while he brushed his teeth, so he didn't notice.

The products I use are as natural as possible. On a non-wash day, I've got a spray bottle of water mixed with a little rosemary oil that I've made myself. I spray this on Roman's wet hair and comb it from the bottom up to limit damage. I get a small blob of conditioner and run it through the ends, and use my fingers to gently separate the curls. I always let Roman's hair dry naturally and never use a towel. I used to worry about leaving his hair wet and going out, but it's never been a problem. When I pick him up from school his curls are perfect. I try not to tie his hair back too much as it ruins his curls.

He defines his whole look by his curls. When he says, 'I want to look like Roman,' he pulls his curls over his face.

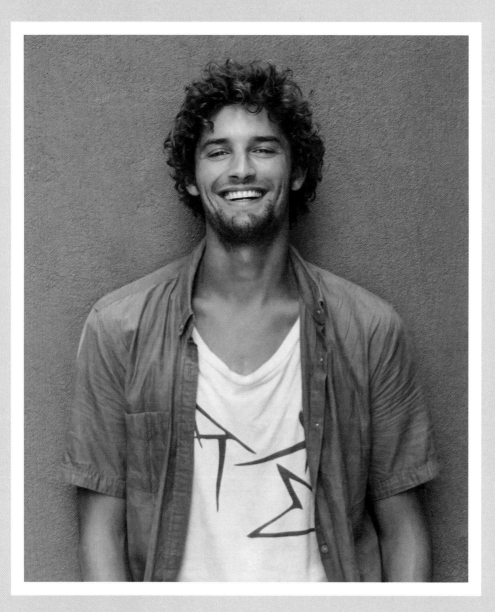

Men

—

Men need to take care of their curls too!
A few extra tricks make all the difference.

Fundamentally, the principles for curly-haired men are the same as for women. Many guys try to shear their curls completely to avoid dealing with them, but they are missing out.

A generalisation about men that is sometimes true is that they tend to spend less money and time on their hair than women. But saving a few pennies on a haircut might mean that you pay the price of a terrible look that will take weeks to grow out. You absolutely can find a good barber at an affordable price – just make sure that they are experienced with curly hair so you don't have to worry about them going wild with the clippers.

Men are also more prone to hair loss than women. Follow the tips in this book on gentle drying (pages 42–47), minimal shampoo use (page 30) and using the right tools, combs and brushes (pages 77–83) to ensure that your hair stays strong and healthy. Growing out your curls will also give your hair the appearance of being thicker and fuller. Look after your curls and your future self will thank you!

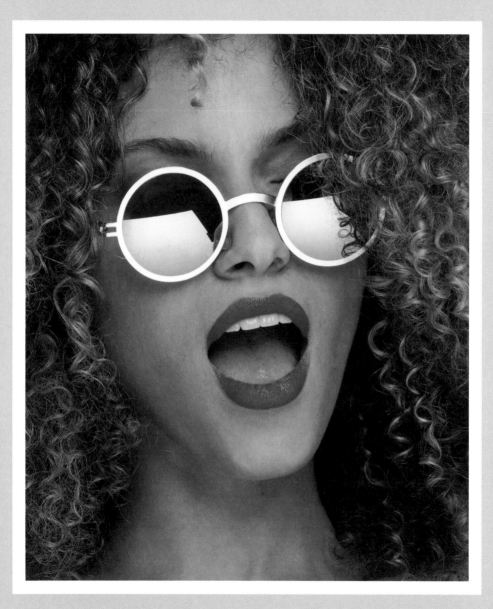

Summer hair

Summer has its own challenges when it comes to
caring for curls. Spending time outdoors in
the sun and possibly the sea takes its toll on hair,
making it drier and more difficult to manage.

Compensate for any summer damage by using a mild shampoo and never shirking on conditioner – a cleansing conditioner that contains essential oils will wash your hair without stripping it like a shampoo will.

In addition, avoid hairdryers and other heat-utilising styling products or, at least, turn the temperature right down. Alternatively, opt to dry your hair naturally during the warmer months; your curls will thank you for it.

A sunburnt scalp is also best avoided: wear a hat! If you do fall victim, avocado can be a great, natural solution, and it's the basis of the scalp-restoring hair mask on page 101. It will also soothe your sore head. Follow this with a gently exfoliating hair mask, which will remove dead skin while also sealing in moisture. Lather this up in place of your regular shampoo, rinsing well afterwards, and then allow your hair to dry naturally. Your healthy, beachy curls will be the perfect holiday accessory.

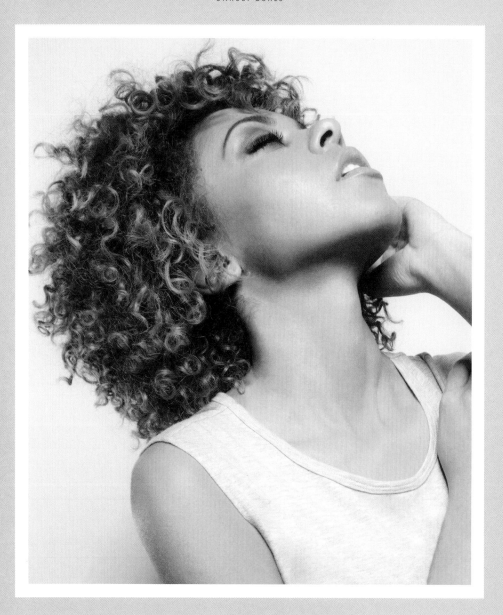

100

Summer hair make-at-home treatments

STYLING WITH SALT SPRAY

Enhance your summer look with your own customised salt spray. You'll need a spray bottle for your beach-perfect creation.

✳ Ingredients
1 cup (240 ml/8 fl oz) hot water
1–2 tsp sea salt (more for a beachier look)
1 tbsp coconut oil, argan oil, or ½ of each (we like using both!)
½ tsp leave-in conditioner
dab of pomade or water-based gel

✳ Method
1. Add the water to the spray bottle.
2. Add the ingredients and shake for about a minute.
3. Spray liberally onto towel-dried hair and scrunch, scrunch, scrunch with your hands.
4. Plait your hair in a loose braid or pile it on top of your head in a loose knot while it dries. When it's almost dry, let your hair down, scrunch some more, then leave it to dry completely naturally. Enjoy those beautifully defined curls.

SCALP-RESTORING HAIR MASK

The saturated fats, vitamins A and E, protein and various other minerals in avocado are highly beneficial for dry and damaged hair, and will help add moisture to dry hair shafts and strengthen your hair.

✳ Ingredients
1 ripe avocado, peeled and stoned
1 teaspoon wheatgerm oil
1 teaspoon jojoba oil

✳ Method
1. Mash the avocado in a bowl. Mix in the oils to make a smooth paste.
2. Apply the mixture to freshly washed hair, from the roots to the ends. Cover your hair with a shower cap, leave it on for an hour and then shampoo your hair with lukewarm water. Use when your curls need revitalising.

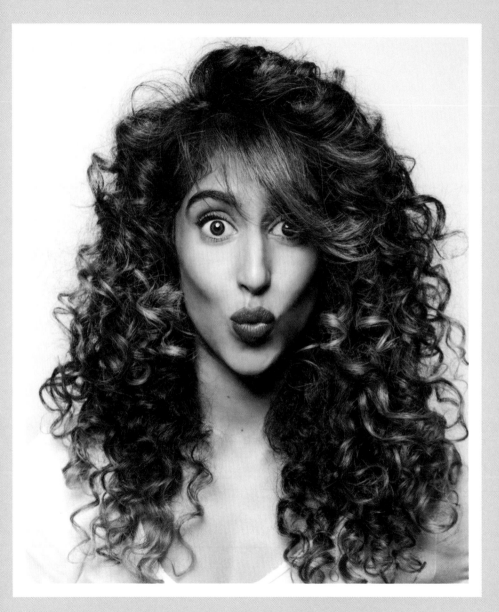

Festival hair

———

Quick-fix festival hair hacks for curly hair are worth knowing, particularly because you may not be able to wash and condition your hair as you usually would.

✳ Work a water-based, weightless texture spray onto your palms and into your hair. Run your hands over your curls, scrunching from the ends up to the roots.

✳ Flip your head forward and scrunch up the tips of your hair all the way up to your roots.

✳ Finally, rub your fingers at the scalp to create lift and volume, fluffing up your curls.

✳ Mix water with a leave-in conditioner and spray throughout your hair.

✳ At festivals, dry shampoo will become your best friend!

✳ Always have a hairband on your wrist. Perfect for whipping your hair into an emergency topknot when things have gone a bit wild and it looks unmanageable.

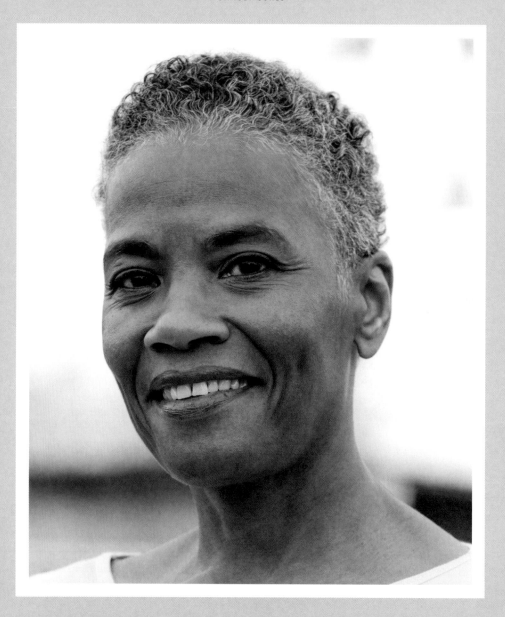

Grey hair

—

We aren't going to spout on about how age is just a number, because you already know that. What we believe is that whatever your age, whether male or female, you can make your grey curls your strongest fashion statement with a bit of thought and care.

105

CUT It is essential to trim your hair every 6-8 weeks for easier manageability and healthier hair; this will immediately pay dividends.

SHAMPOO Grey hair is vulnerable to breakage as it is usually finer and not as well-moisturised due to decreased sebum production. Protect against this with a hydrating shampoo which helps protect grey hairs from becoming brittle.

CONDITION If your hair is naturally curly and grey your hair will need an extra hand in moisturising, because grey hair typically has a coarse, more brittle texture than pigmented hair. Conditioners with natural oils, like argan oil, help lock in moisture and will maintain your curly hair's natural balance.

DEEP CONDITION A weekly deep condition can help keep your curly hair looking good. I recommend liberally applying organic coconut oil to your hair once a week to restore the moisture that is lost along with the pigment when your hair goes grey. Keep the oil on your hair for as long as possible, preferably overnight. Massage a mild shampoo into your hair before rinsing, then leave to dry naturally.

TONE Grey hair can turn yellow and brassy because of external environmental factors like pollution, smoking and even the wrong shampoo. For bright and sparkly silver hair, use a subtly cool-hued toner to give your hair a cool sheen and help offset any yellowing that may occur. The days of the blue rinse are over!

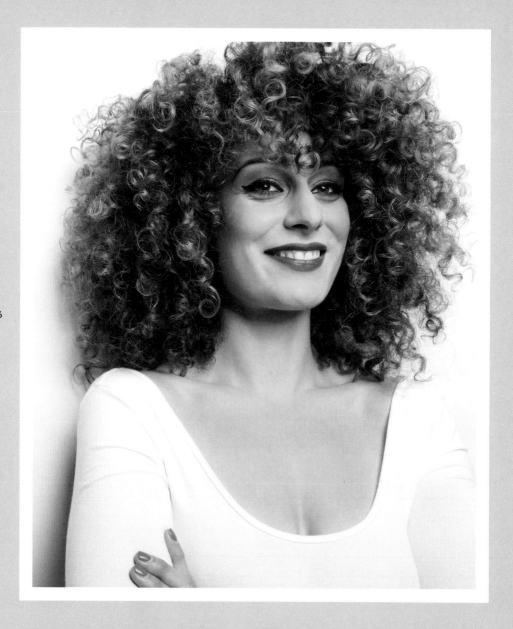

Final thoughts

Most people with curly hair struggle with the same issues: getting a good shape, fighting the frizz and choosing the right products and tools. This book should hopefully have eased these worries and given you renewed confidence so that your curls feel like a blessing instead of a curse.

Learning to care for your hair and how to style it is going to make a huge difference. Perhaps the greatest difference of all will be accepting your hair and learning to love it. Curly hair is an asset and a defining feature to be celebrated. Don't fall into the all too common vicious cycle of not taking the time to find a good stylist, getting a bad cut, then avoiding future haircuts. Take the time to research a good hairdresser for curly hair and talk to them, then work hard on developing a relationship. A good hairdresser will always listen to you. A great hairdresser will take the time to explain what they intend to do and why.

Enjoy those unruly curls!

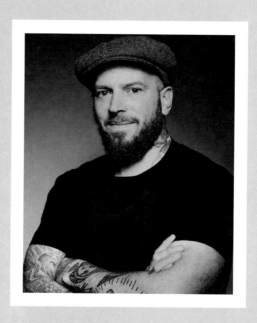

About the author

_____

Michael Price began hairdressing as a Saturday job aged 15 while still at school. He has worked in London since he was 17 and opened the Unruly Curls salon in 2005, catering to and specialising in curly hair.

Michael has also worked as a session stylist, doing hair for TV, film and photography. His techniques with curly hair are mostly self-taught, devised while figuring out the shortcomings in his traditional hairdressing training. He enjoys sharing his knowledge of curly hair and strives to impact a positive change in the way it is understood and appreciated.

In addition to his passion of hairdressing he also enjoys a second career as a photographer.

He lives in Notting Hill with his wife Natasha and two children, George and Theodora.

Instagram: @unrulycurls
Twitter: @wedocurls
Facebook: Unruly Curls London

Thank yous

———

I am forever indebted to my wife, Natasha Devedlaka. Her support throughout my career and her understanding of the long hours and hardships of starting and running a business has been more than I could ever ask or expect.

I am grateful to every person that has ever sat in my chair. I have learned more through them than college or apprenticeships ever taught me.

I would like to make an enormous thanks to Greg Morgan, who gave me my first opportunity in hairdressing, a dear and special character whom I will never forget. Greg took a chance on hiring me and later fired me (I was a wild teen at the time). I remember begging him to reconsider; he did, and I am eternally grateful.

Special thanks to Peter Woodall and Sophie Schreiber who gave me my first job in London.

I am forever grateful to Andrew Edells for his support as I transitioned from a newbie cutter to an experienced professional.

I am thankful to Alba, a client and friend whose way of drying her hair changed the way I work.

A very special thanks to Kate Pollard and my publishers Hardie Grant.

I am forever thankful to Sara Warren for teaching me to apply colour and understand layering. Her support and friendship will never be forgotten.

I am thankful to Victoria Franklin, whose partnership in business I could have not done without.

This book would never have been written without the help of my oldest and dearest friend Clive Philips, who made sense of my curly ramblings.

Unruly Curls would not have ever been had it not been for two very special people in my life – France and Michelangelo Chiacchio who encouraged me from day one of my journey.

My deepest thanks to all of the fantastic team that have worked alongside me at Unruly over the past decade.

Lastly, but most importantly, I am thankful to my children, George and Theodora. They are what drives me to work hard; every moment with them is cherished, and it is for them I do all I do.

Stockists

Shampoo	Conditioner	Styling Products	Tools
Aesop Colour Protection Shampoo www.aesop.com	**Aesop** Colour Protection Conditioner www.aesop.com	**Aveda** Be Curly Enhancing Lotion www.aveda.com	**Fransen** Universal Diffuser www.salonsdirect.co.uk
Cantu Sulphate-Free Cleansing Cream Shampoo www.cantubeauty.com	**Cantu** Sulphate-Free Hydrating Cream Conditioner www.cantubeauty.com	**Boots** Boots Essentials Curl Cream www.boots.com	**Parlux** Superturbo 3000 Hairdryer www.parlux.co.uk www.parluxus.com
Yes To Yes To Carrots Shampoo www.yesto.co.uk www.yesto.com	**Shea Moisture Jamaican** Black Castor Oil Strengthen & Restore Treatment Masque www.boots.com www.sheamoisture.com	**TIGI Catwalk** Curls Rock Amplifier www.allbeauty.com	
	Yes To Yes To Carrots Conditioner www.yesto.co.uk www.yesto.com		

Unruly Curls by Michael Price

First published in 2017 by Hardie Grant Books

Hardie Grant Books (UK)
52-54 Southwark Street
London SE1 1UN
hardiegrant.co.uk

Hardie Grant Books (Australia)
Ground Floor, Building 1
658 Church Street
Melbourne, VIC 3121
hardiegrant.com.au

British Library Cataloguing-in-Publication Data. A catalogue record for this book is available from the British Library.

ISBN: 978-1-78488-082-8

Publisher: Kate Pollard
Senior Editor: Kajal Mistry
Editorial Assistant: Hannah Roberts
Photographer: Michael Price
Art Direction: Daisy Dudley
Copy Editor: Harriet Griffey
Colour Reproduction by p2d

Printed and bound in China by 1010

10 9 8 7 6 5 4 3 2 1